Praise for **HOW TO BE WELL**

"*How to Be Well* is a tour de force of truth when it comes to taking control of your own health and staying well. Health is not something you find in a doctor's office; it's a product of what you think and do every day. Let this book be your guide."

—**CHRISTIANE NORTHRUP, MD,** *New York Times* best-selling author of *Goddesses Never Age*

"*How to Be Well* is the last book you will need to buy if you follow its simple, clear, powerful advice on how to create health. Dr. Frank Lipman has made over 30 years of experience in healing patients into a fun, enlightening, practical guide for being well."

—**MARK HYMAN, MD,** Director, Cleveland Clinic Center for Functional Medicine, and #1 *New York Times* best-selling author of *Food: What the Heck Should I Eat?*

"*How to Be Well* is exactly what it says: an essential manual for thriving in the modern world. Frank Lipman has been my trusted well-being doctor, and now everybody can have access to his insight on the keys to living a healthy, vibrant life. It should be on every nightstand." —**ARIANNA HUFFINGTON**

"Dr. Lipman has done it again (and again). He always inspires me to be a better version of myself by making real lifestyle changes that stick. He educates and motivates by telling us how to get all the benefits of a wellness lifestyle. I'll keep this one close by—everyone should!" —**BOBBI BROWN**

"As a practicing physician trained in Western and Eastern medicine, Dr. Lipman has deep experience in the challenges of maintaining wellness today. In *How to Be Well,* he provides a holistic recipe for health. Use this book as an antidote to the toxic modern environment." —**DAVID LUDWIG, MD, PhD,** Professor, Harvard Medical School, and author of #1 *New York Times* bestseller, *Always Hungry? Conquer Cravings, Retrain Your Fat Cells, and Lose Weight Permanently*

"The guidance Dr. Lipman presents is at once deceptively simple and yet profoundly elegant and universally true. These are the very answers that will allow your body to unlock its own innate healing capacity to prevent and reverse chronic disease so that you not only have many years in your life, but much life in your years." —**AVIVA ROMM, MD,** author of *The Adrenal Thyroid Revolution*

"Dr. Lipman is one of the true pioneers in integrative medicine, preaching and practicing it long before it became 'cool.' In *How to Be Well,* he condenses his 30 years of experience into simple steps to achieve the holy grail: wellness. You could not ask for a better guide on your journey to health. Read and follow this book!" —**STEVEN R. GUNDRY, MD,** *New York Times* best-selling author of *The Plant Paradox* and *The Plant Paradox Cookbook,* and Medical Director, The Centers for Restorative Medicine

HOW TO
BE WELL

For information about permission to
reproduce selections from this book, write to
trade.permissions@hmhco.com or to Permissions,
Houghton Mifflin Harcourt Publishing Company,
3 Park Avenue, 19th Floor, New York, New York 10016.

hmhco.com

*Library of Congress Cataloging-in-Publication Data is
available.*
ISBN 978-1-328-90478-2 (hardcover)
ISBN 978-1-328-90507-9 (ebook)

Book design by PG&Co
Illustrations by Giacomo Bagnara

Printed in the United States of America
DOC 10 9 8 7 6 5 4 3 2 1

HOW TO BE WELL

The Six Keys to a Happy and Healthy Life

FRANK LIPMAN, MD
WITH AMELY GREEVEN

Houghton Mifflin Harcourt

Boston New York 2018

CONTENTS

UNWIND

CONNECT

WHAT TO DO WHEN . . .

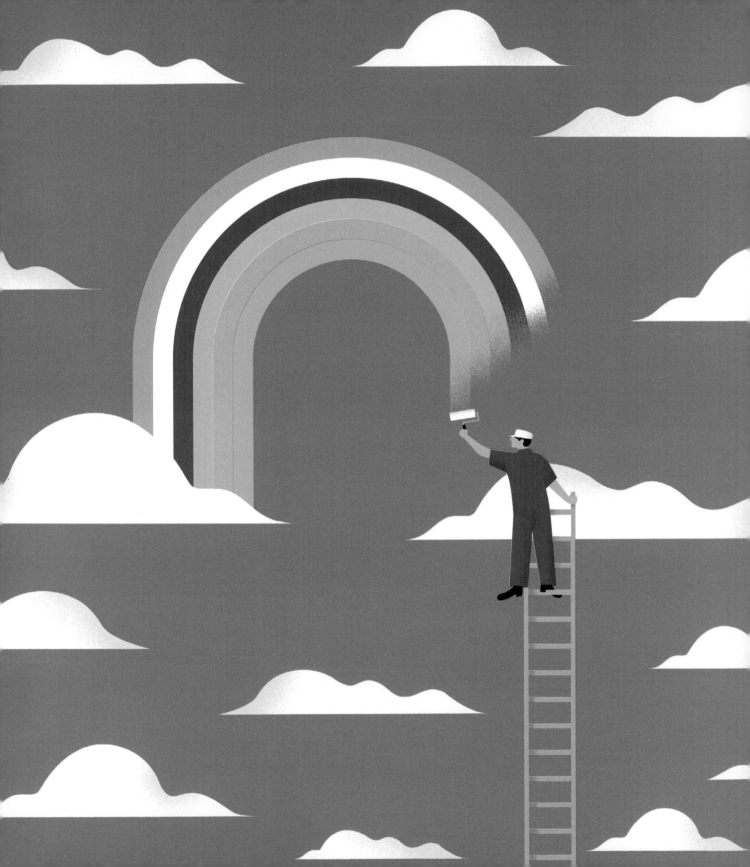

INTRODUCTION

YOU ARE HOLDING IN YOUR HANDS A FIELD GUIDE TO BEING WELL IN AN INCREASINGLY UNWELL WORLD. THIS BOOK IS A LITTLE DIFFERENT FROM OTHER HEALTH BOOKS OUT THERE. IN ITS PAGES YOU WON'T FIND A STRICT DOCTRINE ON DIET OR A SPARTAN THREE-WEEK BOOT CAMP FOR INSTANT TRANSFORMATION. INSTEAD, THIS

IS A HANDBOOK FILLED WITH THE EVERYDAY HABITS and practices you can deploy to launch a healthy lifestyle—or to sustain it, or even master it, depending on where you are starting from and your level of expertise. Just like a wilderness guide is used by novice and seasoned nature-lovers alike—the first-timer needs tips on erecting a tent, the pro needs a primer on rappelling—*How to Be Well* is a manual of the essential skills that anyone can use to navigate safely and smoothly through the wild terrain of wellness today. It is designed to accompany you on the journey of your life and become dog-eared with use.

And it *is* a wild world we find ourselves in today. I have been a doctor for more than thirty-five years, and never have I seen people feeling as tired and sick, at such young ages, as I see now. I have never felt such a surge of profit-driven interests—Big Food, Big Pharma, and Big Tech—shaping the ways we eat, think, and treat our bodies and minds. In addition, the number of brands and products promising to deliver better health is dizzying. If you are a health-seeker, finding your way through this crowded landscape of information, misinformation, and glittering promise can feel disorienting. You might want to take the right steps to stay well and energized and avoid the decline you are being told is inevitable as you age. You might want to resolve chronic symptoms, or get a handle on weight issues, or better your state of mind. But knowing

the direction to start walking can be confounding, and having the time or energy to figure it out in the midst of a busy life—who has that? More and more, my patients want less talk and more action. They say, "*Just tell me what I need to do!*"

What I've observed is that the people who are most successful at achieving—and then maintaining—a healthy lifestyle, and who have the highest levels of vitality, resilience, and longevity, have found their way through this landscape thanks to two things: They have guides and mentors they turn to who give them the information and inspiration they need to adopt small, meaningful habits. And they make change—according to their own needs, interests, and natures, incrementally building their strong and long-lasting house of health.

How to Be Well is designed to give you the same ongoing guidance. Its purpose is simple: to help you build and maintain your resilient house of health, one that can weather the storms of modern living, that you enjoy inhabiting, and that is uniquely your own, constructed your way. In an era when many people say their primary care provider wouldn't recognize them on the street, this book exists to put responsibility and power firmly into your own hands. Today, more than any time in recent decades, the primary care provider is you.

THE GOOD MEDICINE PHILOSOPHY

BEFORE WE GO ANY FARTHER, LET'S THINK POSITIVE. DESPITE THE ALARMING STATE OF CHRONIC ILLNESS IN AMERICA (AND MOST OTHER INDUSTRIALIZED NATIONS), DESPITE THE VERY ROCKY AND VULNERABLE STATE OF OUR HEALTHCARE SYSTEM AND THE PREVAILING—AND BANK-BREAKING—NOTION THAT "MORE MEDICINE IS

BETTER" WHEN IT COMES TO FIXING PROBLEMS, WE are actually in the middle of a revolution. We are waking up to the much bigger and broader picture of how to be well, and that is what you will find in this book. I began my career as a traditionally trained MD in my native South Africa, then studied Chinese medicine in the U.S. I became an adopter of functional medicine and was an early practitioner of implementing gut repair and detoxification to address two frequent root causes of illness, which were getting overlooked. Today those components merge under an umbrella that I officially term "integrative medicine," but what I mainly call, quite simply, *Good Medicine.*

Good Medicine uses a wide and inclusive aperture to look at the state of your body and mind, and it looks for fundamental causes of weakness and imbalance before throwing drugs and medical interventions at a problem. It asks lots of questions: What are you eating? How are you sleeping? Do you wake up each day raring to go? How sedentary is your work day? Who cares about you, and how do you feel when you're alone? The elements that either create good health or deplete it are largely the very ordinary parts of life—our food, rhythms, environment, and relationships—and they all interrelate, all the time. Health or disease is almost always multifactorial in cause and is typically the outcome of the small choices you make daily: You can eat the most pristine diet in the world, but if you're wound as tight as a drum or feel cut off from support, or you exercise until you drop each day, the easeful well-being you desire can elude you.

Good Medicine also sees health as a fluid entity, not a fixed state. That means that what works for you today might not work so well in five or ten years. Change is constant when it comes to your physical and mental state, and the way to ride those waves, and to truly be well, is to know yourself well. Good Medicine views you as an individual, the owner of a unique constitution metabolically, psychologically, and emotionally, not a one-size-fits-all machine that thrives on hard-and-fast rules. While there certainly are universal laws that apply to everyone with a human design—eating lots of vegetables is nonnegotiable for nourishment, detoxification, and disease prevention, and sleep is essential for healing and repair—how *you* choose to implement those habits is a personal matter. Spinach or cauliflower; night owl or lark; rock climber or swimmer— you need to pick what works for your needs, tendencies, and tolerances so you can establish the habits that work for you and succeed at maintaining them. Furthermore, your physiological needs and personal preferences shift at different phases of your life or in response to changing circumstances.

What this all means is that to truly be well, *you* need to know *you*. Which is why *How to Be Well* is designed to make you the author of your health story. It does this by ditching the linear "follow this program" approach that insists that every single person must do the same sequence of step A, then step B, then C, and that focuses on only one aspect of wellness. Instead, it offers you a new map for a new medicine, one that is not linear at all but circular.

A DEEPER LOOK AT GOOD MEDICINE

THERE ARE THREE BIG GOALS OF GOOD MEDICINE, AND THEY FORM THE PHILOSOPHICAL BACKBONE for all the advice in this book:

RESILIENCE

You cannot guarantee that you won't ever meet germs, viruses, toxins, mean people, and hard times. How well you face these obstacles and how easily you bounce back is determined by resilience. The gift of resilience is that it gives you a solid and very seaworthy ship, so that when a storm comes, you don't drown. When resilience is optimized, you can handle temporary and unexpected changes a little better. When resilience is depleted, you are much more vulnerable: You crumble when you get a cold and can get easily unraveled by psychological stressors. It's a total-sum game: When one piece of the puzzle, like sleep or good diet, gets off track, you can get off track. Resilience is a quality you can build through simple lifestyle choices.

FUNCTION

Where Western medicine often approaches health with "you're fine until the day you are not," Good Medicine does not see "health" and "illness" as polar extremes. Instead, it sees a spectrum ranging from less optimal to highly optimal, with vitality, resilience, and positive mindset increasing or diminishing depending on where on the spectrum you are. When you take care to improve the function of your organs and systems before any weakness takes hold and notice early if you backslide, you can correct any imbalance before it becomes a disease. The keys to optimizing function are paying attention to changes as they are happening instead of powering past them, and being willing to inves-tigate the deeper causes of symptoms rather than automatically suppressing them with medication to make them go away. It's reassuring when you use this spectrum as your framework for health. Even if you've indulged in years of hard living, you can mobilize yourself to get to the brighter end of the spectrum.

SYNERGY

Synergy refers to the "extra" you get when several different elements, such as the various organs and systems of the body, are working together. You can have positive synergy, in which every positive change creates more positive changes, or you can have negative synergy, in which every dysfunction creates more and more dysfunction. Good health comes from harnessing the power of positive synergy through fairly modest actions and everyday habits. Resetting your sleep rhythms, plus getting out into nature, plus spending time with a friend who listens to you, can reduce a cortisol storm initiated by stress. This gives your adrenals and thyroid a break, which improves digestive function and allevi-ates brain fog, restores a regular menstrual cycle or sex drive, helps your body burn calories efficiently, improves self-esteem, and ignites a desire to enroll in a strength-training class . . . it's a ripple effect. Synergy is the reason the small, ordinary things we often take for granted can catalyze extraordinary improvements in health and happiness. *How to Be Well* is built on the concept of this ripple effect—the Six Rings of Good Medicine even look like ripples on the surface of a pond.

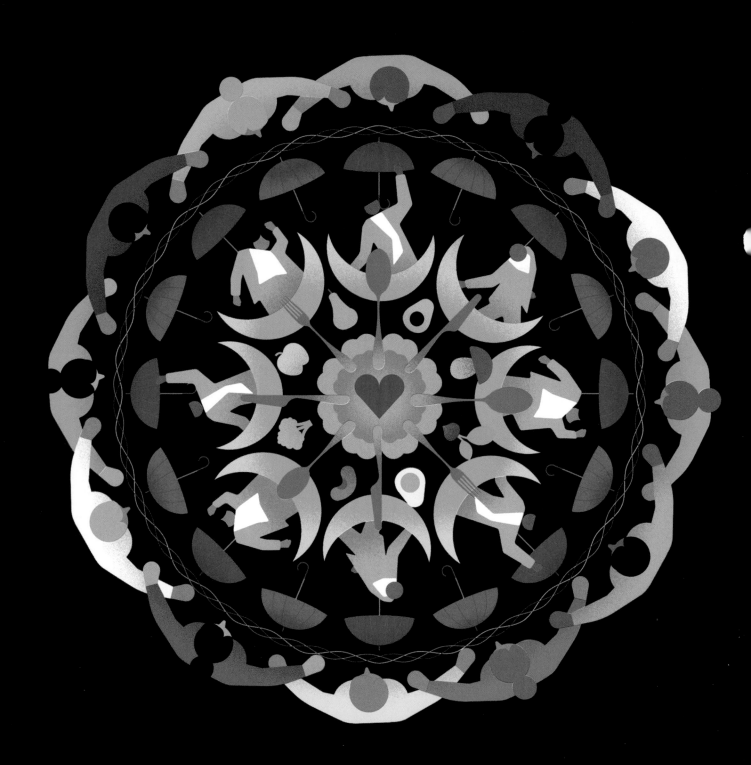

THE GOOD MEDICINE MANDALA

THE GOOD MEDICINE MANDALA IS A CIRCULAR SYSTEM IN WHICH YOU, NOT A DOCTOR OR ANY OTHER AUTHORITY FIGURE, STAND AT THE CENTER. SIX RINGS SURROUND YOU, REPRESENTING THE SIX SPHERES OF LIFE THAT I KNOW TO BE THE PILLARS OF LONG-LASTING HEALTH. WHEN YOU RESTORE OR OPTIMIZE ALL THESE SPHERES, YOU WILL LEAD THE PACK IN TERMS OF YOUR STANDARD OF HEALTH AND ENJOYMENT OF LIFE.

The Six Rings of Good Medicine ripple outward from the most material aspect of health—the food you eat—to the subtlest one, which is your sense of connection to the world at large.

MOVING FROM THE INNER RING AT THE CENTER OUTWARD, THE SIX RINGS ARE:

HOW TO EAT	MASTERING THE VERY BUILDING BLOCKS OF LIFE—FOOD.
HOW TO SLEEP	REPRIORITIZING AND RESTORING ONE OF YOUR MOST FUNDAMENTAL NEEDS.
HOW TO MOVE	ENSURING THE BODY MOVES IN ALL THE WAYS THAT NATURE INTENDED IT TO.
HOW TO PROTECT	MITIGATING AND PREVENTING THE INVISIBLE ASSAULT OF EVERYDAY TOXINS.
HOW TO UNWIND	CONSCIOUSLY SWITCHING OFF TO ALLOW FOR COMPLETE MENTAL AND PHYSIOLOGICAL REPRIEVE.
HOW TO CONNECT	AWAKENING AND ENHANCING A SENSE OF BELONGING AND MEANING.

Each of the six rings contains the blueprints or instructions for a range of small actions you can take to improve and strengthen your levels of resilience and functioning. Some of these instructions are long because they cover a significant new habit, like building physical strength or restoring your body's sleep clock. Others are simply a nugget—a small idea for you to chew on and try when you have a few moments of free time.

You can decide which actions in *How to Be Well* to try depending on how you work best and how much time, energy, or bandwidth for newness you have available. Some people like to dive into one area of wellness, such as nutrition, and do a clean sweep there before attending to another area like physical fitness or stress reduction. If that's you, start with the How to Eat ring and explore it deeply, picking out the actions you want to try (see How to Use This Book, opposite) and working through as many as you feel called to do. If that's not you, use the book more spontaneously: Let your eye land on something that speaks to you, try that habit, and get in a groove with it gradually before you open the book again. Because all the actions positively influence one another—for example, meditation tends to help you fall asleep earlier, and better sleep helps reduce cravings for sugar—it doesn't matter where you start and in which order you proceed. And take as long as you need: Spend a few weeks or (ideally) a few months! Just don't try to make too many changes at once. What I've found in watching patients improve their health is that there is a common pattern to becoming well: One small success, and one happily engrained new habit, paves the way for the next. Slow and steady wins the race, because with each healthy change, you win back some energy and clarity and gain confidence in your abilities and enthusiasm, which powers you to the next healthy habit. What science tells us is that once a habit is developed, it works effortlessly for you, partly because the brain *loves* habits. When lifestyle choices become habitual, they are automatic. This frees up energy for the brain to focus on more meaningful things—like problem-solving and creativity—and helps override the urges toward negative habits.

The inspiration for the Good Medicine Mandala came from my clinical experience working with patients and observing what helps them make—and stick to—positive, health-giving changes. The efforts of my amazing team of health coaches at my practice, the Eleven Eleven Wellness Center in New York City, are partly to thank for this. They guide my patients to make the positive changes that I suggest—they don't push, bully, judge, or focus on things that are out of reach. They simply ask each patient "What do you think *you* can do today?" to help break down the goal of better health into bite-size chunks: *For breakfast, cut out the cereal and have some eggs. Take a ten-minute walk. Take three deep breaths before getting out of bed. Attend a women's circle on Friday night.* This level of personalization and practicality leads to success because that single new habit often leads to a widespread lifestyle upgrade.

In case you are wondering what a mandala is, it's a visual tool used in meditation to help focus your mind and bring awareness and order to every part of your self: body, mind, and spirit. I've adopted it as an organizing principle for a collection of simple habits, actions, and practices that you can use to improve and maintain your level of wellness. It is also a symbol to remind you that everything you learn about your health is actually—ultimately—about learning fully and profoundly about *you*. This is why "you" sit at the very center of the six rings.

The Good Medicine Mandala may resemble an archery target to you, with a bull's-eye at its center. That's a good interpretation: A target helps you focus your aim and is an instrument for practicing your skills. Your arrow may land on one ring today and another ring tomorrow; where you take aim is up to you. The mandala may also strike you as the rings of a tree trunk, which form as the tree grows. The process of creating better health grows in depth and meaning as you mature, and the challenges we face often lead to wisdom and inner strength. And if it looks like a ripple on a pond spreading outward from a dropped pebble—touching one ring and then the next, and ultimately, rippling out farther to the greater field around you—you've read enough to know that beautifully captures the aim of this book.

If it looks a bit like a game, that's also intentional. Some of the best healers in the world use playfulness as a primary strategy because it helps you get past fear and fire up belief in your body's innate power to heal.

>> **Health is the outcome of the small choices you make on a daily basis.** <<

HOW TO USE THIS BOOK

Begin anywhere you like. If concrete actions like eating more vegetables (page 58) are easier to start with than investing in friendship (page 230), start at the first ring of the Mandala, How to Eat, and pick several actions or practices to focus on for the coming weeks. Some are things you can practice for a few days or a week, while others, like quitting sugar or switching to a low-carb diet, are lifestyle changes that may take longer to fully engrain. Then, when you are ready for another practice, pick another page to look at. When you have completed as many actions from the How to Eat ring as you want to do, move to the next ring, How to Sleep, and pick a few actions that resonate with your needs. Keep moving from ring to ring, gradually working your way out to the subtler zones of connection and creativity and purpose.

If you'd rather use this book in a "choose your own adventure" kind of way, page through it and pick the first thing that pops out as inspiring and interesting. Master that—if you like, make a note of what you did—then page through again, charting a more eclectic path. There is no minimum or maximum number of actions to take; you will benefit even if you try only one thing from each ring. However, my hope is that you spend time becoming "habitual" with many actions in every ring—and that you use this book over the long term, gradually acquiring new habits as your life allows.

To keep track of your work, you can use one of the Be Well action charts available to download at howtobewell.com. You can use these to plot out which actions you want to try over the next one, two, three months and more, to provide a level of accountability and support your commitment. You can even team up with others to map out a path using the Good Medicine Mandala that you will do together. Whichever way you use this book, you will engage in a continuum of progress that is doable, fun, and deeply meaningful.

In addition to the action charts, howtobewell.com provides extra content that makes the instructions found in these pages come to life. As you read, look for callouts that direct you to videos, charts, and other supporting material.

THE HOW TO BE WELL PROS

AS YOU MOVE THROUGH THE MANDALA, YOU WILL DISCOVER INSIGHTS AND ADVICE from the specialists I rely on to guide my patients in areas outside my own expertise. These are not the ones in white coats (though I would certainly call on them if an acute situation required it). These specialists are the leading voices in their respective fields of fitness, meditation, clean eating, self-fulfillment, and more. I dub them the Be Well Pros, and they share strategies and tactics that will help you not only establish your new normal but truly get to your A game.

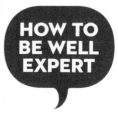
HOW TO BE WELL EXPERT

THE FOUR DIRECTIONS

I CREATED THE MANDALA WITH FOUR SPECIFIC HEALTH FACTORS IN MIND. THESE LIE UNDER, AND ALSO CON-
NECT, MANY OF THE ACTIONS IN THE RINGS, LIKE FOUR POINTS ON THE COMPASS. I WANT YOU TO BECOME
MORE AWARE OF THESE FACTORS AS YOU MAKE CHOICES ABOUT HOW YOU EAT, SLEEP, AND TAKE CARE OF

YOURSELF EACH DAY, BECAUSE THEY ARE COMMON areas of dysfunction that have the power to shape how you feel, perform, think, heal, and age. You'll see them referred to numerous times throughout the rings, and after spending some time with this book, you will become knowledgeable about how and where they tend to get unbalanced and why that has such an effect on your health.

When you are familiar with the Four Directions, you will also feel more sure-footed about *why* you are making the positive changes. This can be very motivating, because the thing about small, meaningful lifestyle changes is that they don't always trigger fireworks and dramatic epiphanies. They are often incremental and cause shifts at a realistic, yet moderate pace. An understanding of these foundational principles will help you stay on course when you feel an urge to drink the corn-syrup-laden soda for energy or surf the web in the wee hours when you should be sleeping.

THE FOUR DIRECTIONS ARE:

YOUR MICROBIOME Perhaps the most studied and talked-about area of health today, the thriving communities of various viruses, bacteria, fungi, and protozoa known collectively as your microbiome reside in vast numbers in your gut as well as on your skin, in your mouth, and in other body parts. In the old days, when I first began practicing medicine, doctors thought of this biome as merely comprising various organisms assisting in digestion; decades later, we know it's much more complicated and that the microbiome has the power to impact almost every area of your health, including your immunity, stress response, sleep, mood and behavior, metabolism, weight, and so on.

This extraordinarily diverse ecosystem plays many roles: It helps break down food and extract essential nutrients; produces vitamins and brain chemicals; and fends off microbial invaders by "talking to" your natural-killer T cells, protecting you from disease. The microbiome impacts many critical functions that control your metabolism. The diversity and health of these minuscule biota influence the way you use energy or hold on to it in the form of excess weight, and a damaged microbiome can initiate runaway inflammation starting in the gut wall, leading not only to increased intestinal permeability or "leaky gut," but subsequent insulin resistance and fat accumulation. (New research suggests that an underlying cause of obesity may be impaired gut microbiome composition, in part because it alters the brain's signals for fullness.) The resulting systemic inflammation can show up as symptoms anywhere in the body.

That's just the beginning—your microbiome performs hundreds of tasks essential to keeping your systems functioning optimally, including helping you sync up with the natural rhythms of day and night and falling asleep easily, and helping your brain work smoothly and without anxiety. Unfortunately, almost no one reaches adulthood with their microbiome in tip-top shape—it picks up a few dents and dings along the way, from gut-busters like drugs and antibiotics, junk food, GMOs, conventionally or factory-farmed meats, and other assaults on your inner ecology. In order for your immune system, metabolism, inflammatory response, sleep, and brain to function well, protecting your microbiome—and restoring its balance if it is disrupted—is one of the most important things you can do to sustain health.

YOUR INFLAMMATORY RESPONSE The immune system is one of our most brilliantly engineered bodily systems. It is designed to leap into action when the presence of danger is detected—like an invading pathogen or a foreign substance that shouldn't be there—and use emergency measures to tackle and take it out. One of those measures is inflammation, and inflammation serves a powerful purpose when used as an occasional weapon of defense. Today, our systems are so overloaded with small assaults and aggravations, from unnatural foods, to toxins and drugs, to stress and lack of sleep, that the alarm can ring constantly if we don't set up the best possible protection to keep invaders out. Chronic inflammation initiated by lifestyle is often the starting point for diseases that are tragically becoming endemic, such as heart disease, cancer, obesity, arthritis, and many forms of dementia including Alzheimer's. It can be tamed, however, first by replacing the sugars, industrial oils, processed foods, and factory-farmed meats with truly wholesome real foods—a major focus of the first ring of the Mandala—and taking care of the state of the gut microbiome, and then by employing many of the other lifestyle interventions in the Mandala's next five rings.

YOUR RHYTHMS You are a creature of rhythm, living in a world of rhythms. Your biology is governed by rhythm in ways you barely recognize and is designed to exist in sync with the rhythms of day and night and the seasons. Most people are familiar with the concept of circadian rhythms—just one of many internal clocks that we have—but that familiarity doesn't necessarily breed respect! Our lifestyles try to override these rhythms, disrupting them with eating at all hours of day and night, traveling across time zones, air-conditioning, heating and artificial lighting, food shipped from opposite hemispheres, and more. Things that our parents' and grandparents' generations took for granted—like that planning meals and cooking every day are a nonnegotiable part of life—have come into question in our 24/7, service-oriented culture. We are sold the idea that spontaneity, newness, and unpredictability are prized values—they mean you are creative and innovative! Not so for your body, it turns out, which lives for rhythm and balance.

Falling out of sync with the micro and macro rhythms of life has the effect of feeling like swimming upstream, because all sorts of systems in the body rely on those rhythms to work well. The good news is that you can reset your clocks and restore your rhythms, and the ways to do so may surprise you (page 98).

YOUR BALANCE We've ignored the concept of balance at our peril. First, we've forgotten what ancient systems, such as Chinese and Ayurvedic medicine, knew. A physical

We need to start thinking of the body as an integrated whole, and not as a machine with separate parts treated independently.

symptom is a pointer to something in the body system that is out of balance, not an annoying disruption that must be extinguished at all costs. To resolve the symptom, we typically need to work at the level of restoring balance, usually by removing something that is harming you and restoring something that's lacking. If you simply suppress the symptom with a drug, that imbalance will likely pop up somewhere else in your body, trying to get your attention in another way. Plus, you can get on the downward roller-coaster ride of medication side effects, as one prescription symptom-blocker tends to lead to the next.

It's not surprising that this has happened—our entire culture has tipped out of balance. Through a Chinese medicine perspective, it has become dominated by "yang"—the impulse to do more, go faster, and constantly generate things. This is contributing to a level of exhaustion, an overly "outward" identification with material things, and a level of aggression that is unsustainable. (Sounds quite inflamed, doesn't it?) Understanding and embracing the complementary impulse of "yin"—quiet, inward, deep, still—is essential to bringing yourself back into the center, where you are stable and less easily rocked by the events and circumstances around you.

Science is revealing ever-new information about how the Four Directions interrelate. The chain of cause and effect isn't always crystal clear, but the links are unquestionably there. For example, the condition of the microbiome impacts levels of inflammation; it's also been shown to affect circadian rhythms and thereby affect your sleep (among many other things). On the other hand, getting way out of rhythm by shirking proper sleep throws off the balance of hormone production that exists to maintain a healthy metabolism and immune function that helps to prevent disease, which then negatively impacts the functions of the microbiome. Inflammation that changes the ecosystem of the gut, meanwhile, may be responsible for the rise in colorectal cancer, as cancer-causing pathogens invade what was previously walled off. The Four Directions relate in either positive or negative synergy, although you could also think of it as a domino effect: A change in one of the directions, for better or worse, can alter how the other three directions present themselves, even though you didn't intentionally do anything to cause it.

Protecting your microbiome—and restoring its balance if it is disrupted—is one of the most important things you can do to sustain health.

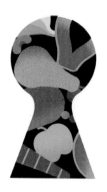

THE TROUBLESHOOTING SECTION

THE IDEA OF SYNERGY COMES INTO PLAY EVEN MORE IN A SECTION OF THE BOOK CALLED "WHAT TO DO WHEN . . . " THIS SECTION PROVIDES INSTRUCTIONS FOR RESOLVING TWELVE OF THE MOST COMMON CHRONIC PROBLEMS I SEE IN MY CLINIC, AND THAT YOU MAY EXPERIENCE YOURSELF. THESE INCLUDE WHAT TO DO WHEN:

. . . **YOU FEEL SLUGGISH AND WANT TO REBOOT**

. . . **YOU WANT TO LOSE WEIGHT**

. . . **YOU ARE FREQUENTLY OVERWHELMED AND ANXIOUS**

. . . **YOU ARE ALWAYS TIRED**

AND SO ON.

In this section you will learn how to address these issues from a Good Medicine approach, integrating habits and actions from each ring to help resolve symptoms at a deeper level than most short doctor visits are able to address. These are not "magic bullet" approaches but programs you can embark on by using the advice in this book. While they may require fine-tuning to hit their ultimate goals, they are the simple "breakthrough tactics" that have aided countless people in resolving troublesome issues and regaining power over their well-being.

My hope is that by using this section as a reference when you feel out of sorts, you will become oriented to the "root-cause" idea of health that underlies my philosophy. To borrow a concept from my Chinese medicine teacher and mentor, Harriet Beinfield, you will begin to "take care of your garden." When you notice a symptom arising that causes discomfort or distress, you won't just blast the leaves of your tree with bug-killers, desperately trying to blitz it away. You'll look a little more calmly, tuning in to find any underlying imbalance in the trunk, then you'll look a little further and detect the cause of that imbalance in the roots. You will water the soil, feed it with super-nutrients, make sure it's getting the right amount of sun, and tend to its entire system wisely. Every one of us has the potential of becoming a wise gardener. And what we find is that the actions wise gardeners take are remarkably consistent—which is why treating many different conditions ultimately comes down to making the same general corrections at this "root" level.

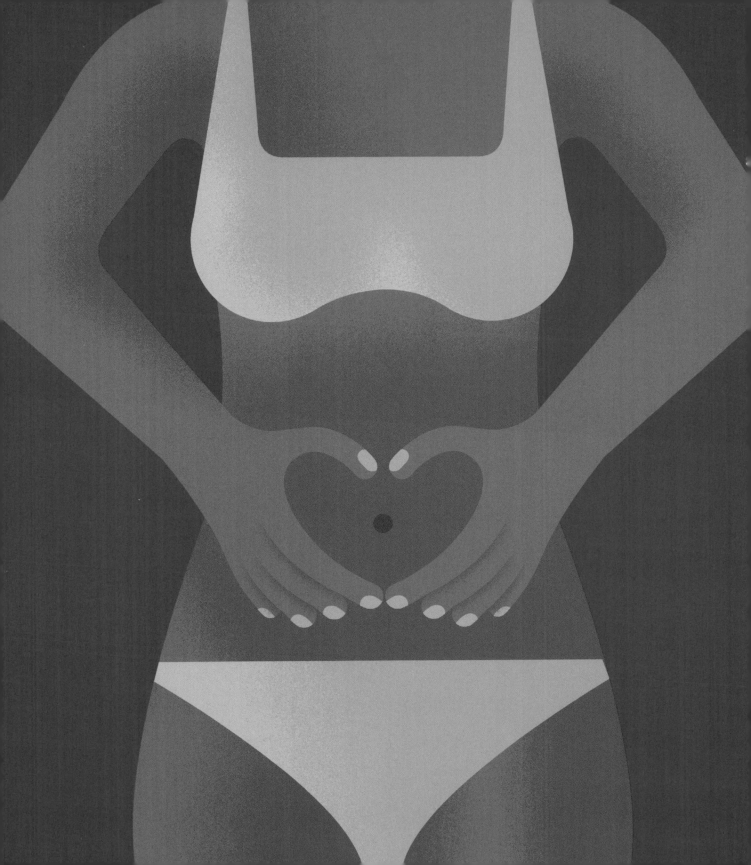

IT STARTS WITH YOU

AFTER YEARS OF PRACTICE, I'VE COME TO KNOW THAT THERE IS NO ONE "RIGHT" WAY TO BE WELL. A DOCTOR OR WELLNESS AUTHORITY CAN OFFER THEIR BEST ASSESSMENT OF THE DIET, ROUTINE, LIFESTYLE, AND MINDSET THEY THINK WILL HELP YOU BEST, BUT YOU INTERPRET THE INFORMATION AND EXPRESS IT IN A COURSE OF ACTION THAT IS UNIQUE TO YOU. ULTIMATELY, THERE is only *your way*.

Establishing your way is a priority for every one of us. Awakening to ourselves also means awakening to the fact that we are living in a world that is out of order. The pressures, the depletions, and the stress that almost all of us live amid are real and they are mounting in intensity, and a gimlet-eyed view will tell you it's not going to stop anytime soon. Our collective reality includes a highly compromised food supply, high-pressure work environments, medication overuse, toxic exposures, social and familial stress, and more. What helps you face these challenges and enjoy your life is knowing what makes you tick and what makes you sick. This comes from learning how to use some fairly simple tools and committing to using them so you can layer in a strong level of resilience and optimal function.

While the project of forging your way forward sounds quite serious—and it is—relax. Rome wasn't built in a day, and robust well-being isn't either. It is a process that starts with a single step, which then leads to another, and another.

One of my mentors in Chinese medicine likes to say that a healing crisis is danger plus opportunity. I believe we are at a collective healing crisis. Though, by all estimations, our average level of health is decreasing (at least it is in the U.S.), there has never been as much collective curiosity, passion, and motivation to live differently. Quality food is easier to find than ever; communities aggregated around healthy living are simpler to locate than before; and solid information from trustworthy sources is getting shared like never before in history. So consider *How to Be Well* an instruction manual for this era of change—a compendium of what you need to know to grab the opportunity in both hands, take "better health" down off the shelf of tomorrows, and start taking steps toward it today.

And why not start right now? When you better your health through even the smallest positive changes, it starts a ripple effect that soon touches others, inspiring and supporting them to make changes, too. That's why a single personal act can have such a meaningful impact: Multiply it by ten, by a hundred, by a thousand other people, and it soon takes on the power to change the world.

>>

Profit-driven interests, like Big Food, Big Pharma, and Big Tech, are shaping the way we eat, think, and treat our bodies and minds. Take back your health.

EAT

THE AMERICAN AUTHOR AND FARMER WENDELL
Berry famously wrote, "People are fed by the food industry, which pays no attention to health, and are treated by the health industry, which pays no attention to food." Most of us would agree the results of this have been disastrous. Luckily, "industrial" eating is no longer the only option. You can forge a more *intimate* relationship with food, demand *integrity* from food, and transform your health completely as a result—food is that powerful.

The actions in this ring promote this intimate relationship. Ask where your food comes from and what happens on the journey from field to fork. Learn if it works for your health or against it (or whether it works for a corporation's bottom line!). And get up close and personal with it every day, preparing meals hands-on whenever possible and experiencing it with all your senses. Be part of the new culture of eating—in which shopping, cooking, and preparing for mealtime is not a stress-inducing burden but something that happens naturally, as part of the rhythm of life.

Industrialized food may have made you fearful about nutrition, and with good reason: Too much of the wrong kinds of food can inflame, aggravate, and exhaust you, and distort the way you feel, think, perform, and heal. But you can turn that angst around with small gains in knowledge (digesting one new dietary teaching at a time), heightened awareness (noticing how foods make you feel), and a few new habits (like taking lunch to work). When you are more intimate with your food, you look at it not as a means to an end—a way not to be hungry!—but as your best ally. And you always ask before you eat it, "What can you do for me today?"

COMPOSE THE **PERFECT PLATE**

IF YOU'VE EVER FRANTICALLY COUNTED CALORIES IN ORDER TO STAY HEALTHY, GIVE YOURSELF A BREAK. PUT THAT EFFORT TOWARD A SIMPLER SYSTEM I CALL THE PERFECT PLATE—A VISUAL PIE CHART THAT GUIDES YOU RIGHT. PICK THE BEST-QUALITY, WHOLE-FOOD INGREDIENTS YOU CAN USING THE GUIDANCE THROUGHOUT

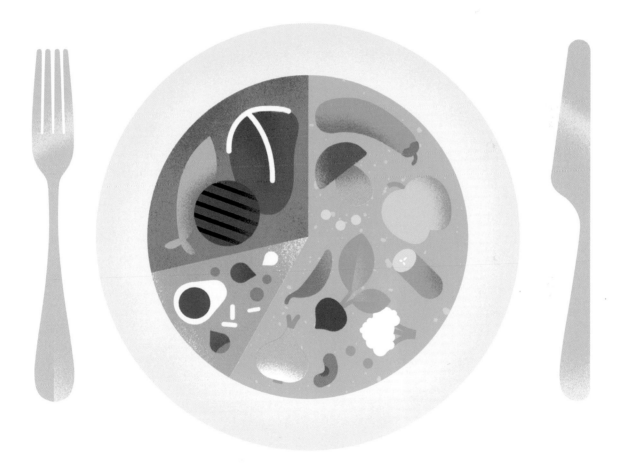

THIS SECTION, THEN COMBINE THEM IN A RATIO THAT gives vegetables the bulk of the plate (or bowl). Make protein a smaller, palm-sized participant, and be sure to add a dose of good fats—either added as a condiment or as part of a fat-rich protein source. The plate should be quite sizeable in volume (from all those vegetables!), but with these proportions in place, you are less likely to

overeat or get out of balance. The Perfect Plate works because it makes you focus on *quality* and not obsess over quantity. By using these health-promoting foods to "crowd out" the bad stuff, it counters what tend to be the real causes of weight dysregulation: too many starches and sugars and inflammatory ingredients, whether from factory-farmed or processed foods.

Use this template to easily put together a great breakfast, lunch, and dinner. (It's a no-rules game: Breakfast can be savory leftovers and dinner can be eggs.) And keep them in mind when ordering meals at restaurants: They will help you custom-create a better meal and remind you to take home part of a supersize protein portion for tomorrow. This simple system teaches you to trust yourself, not a calorie-counting guidebook, to make every meal a boon for your body. If you are following a low-carb protocol (page 85), your plant foods should be mainly nonstarchy vegetables, and for everyone else, I recommend keeping portions of legumes like lentils small and keeping grain portions very small (or nonexistent).

50–70% NON-STARCHY VEGETABLES: (raw, cooked, fermented, sprouted) with fruits and starchy vegetables in moderation. If including other plant foods like legumes, lentils, and grains, keep portion sizes low and, whenever possible, soak and/or sprout them, or use a pressure cooker (page 53), to reduce the inflammatory lectin content and make them more digestible.

10–15% BEST-QUALITY PROTEIN: grass-fed and -finished meats and organic or pastured poultry, wild-caught fish, pasture-raised or organic eggs, organic dairy if tolerated, nuts and seeds, bone broth. If you are vegetarian, modest amounts of legumes like lentils or beans (avoid soy except as a fermented condiment).

20–30% HEALTHY FAT: See Make Friends With Fat, page 30.

TIPS:

- **SOMETIMES YOUR PROTEIN IS FAT-RICH.** Foods like pork, sardines or herring, bacon, chicken with skin, and certain cuts of red meat combine both nutrients.

- **USE SPICES LIBERALLY TO MAKE SIMPLE FOODS POP.**

- **USE LEFTOVERS FROM DINNER FOR BREAKFAST OR LUNCH.**

THE BALANCE OF 3: UNDERSTANDING THE TRIAD

VEGETABLES: Deliver vitamins, nutrients, enzymes, phytonutrients. Give you glowing skin, increase energy, fight cancer, lessen inflammation, increase natural detoxification. Benefit your gut microbiome by adding prebiotics and, if fermented, probiotics.

PROTEIN: Its component amino acids are the building blocks for your body. Gives you strong muscles and immune support.

FAT: Allows you to absorb fat-soluble vitamins and balances hormones. Nourishes your skin, supports your brain, lubricates your digestive system, helps you feel satiated. Can be used as fuel (in the absence of carbohydrates).

- **COOK SEVERAL DAYS' WORTH OF COMPONENTS AHEAD OF TIME,** storing them separately in airtight glass containers in the fridge. Then, for each meal, assemble your plate or bowl, heating to order.

- **GET CREATIVE WITH YOUR PLATE!** Your body and mind love meals that look, smell, and taste appealing. Eat a rainbow of colored vegetables, drizzle and splash healthy oils on top, sprinkle on seeds and nuts.

- **FOLLOW THE GET YOUR VEG TO 70% PRINCIPLES** on page 58.

(EAT THEM FOR BREAKFAST, LUNCH, OR DINNER!)

1 Fried or poached eggs + sautéed spinach + sautéed mushrooms + ghee + avocado

2 Smoothie in a bowl + seeds + berries + cacao nibs + shredded coconut

3 Full-fat grass-fed yogurt + blueberries + seeds

4 Scrambled eggs + buckwheat + guacamole + salsa

5 Paleo bread + avocado + canned wild salmon salad + sprouts

6 Egg muffins + diced tomatoes + mixed greens + EVOO (extra-virgin olive oil)

7 Simple Bone Broth or Vegetable Broth Soup: broth + greens + diced veggies + diced sweet potato + coconut oil

8 Chicken thigh + roasted sweet potato + sautéed broccoli rabe + ghee

9 Smoked salmon + arugula + sliced avocado + sesame seeds + tahini and coconut amino dressing

10 Broiled wild fish + lemon juice + extra-virgin olive oil + roasted broccoli + cauliflower rice

11 Lentil daal + sautéed chard + ghee + full-fat yogurt

12 Lamb burger + steamed dandelion greens with lemon and EVOO + chopped tomatoes + sauerkraut

13 Turkey or beef meatballs + zucchini noodles + pesto or tomato sauce + EVOO

14 Chicken salad (using avocado, not jarred mayo) + chopped romaine lettuce + cherry tomatoes + celery + red onion + hemp seeds + balsamic vinegar + EVOO

15 Roasted beets + roasted sweet potato + roasted Brussels sprouts + arugula + goat cheese

16 Collard Green Wrap: grass-fed beef burger + kimchi + tomato + avocado wrapped in steamed collard greens

17 Broiled or canned sardines + watercress or arugula + EVOO + lemon + olives + capers + fresh herbs

18 Veggie Quinoa Bowl (more veggies/less quinoa): roasted veggies + avocado + pickled veggies

19 Slow-cooked bean or beef stew made with bone broth + steamed greens

20 Sliced grass-fed steak + bed of leafy greens + avocado + portobello mushroom + pumpkin seeds

21 Roasted turkey + cauliflower mash + sautéed kale + EVOO

22 Canned sardines, mixed with lemon and EVOO + olives + capers + diced cucumber + bed of arugula

23 Sushi Roll: smoked/canned salmon + avocado + cucumber + scallion + watercress + cauliflower rice + coconut aminos + sesame seeds wrapped in nori sheet

Liberally use herbs, lemon, sea salt, and garlic to season any plates as you like.

PRACTICE SUGAR
SELF-DEFENSE

SOME AREAS OF NUTRITION HAVE ROOM FOR NEGOTIATION. BUT WHEN IT COMES TO THE SWEET STUFF, THE LINE IS DRAWN. SUGAR IS PUBLIC HEALTH ENEMY NUMBER ONE: THE WORST TOXIN WE EXPOSE OURSELVES TO DAILY IN THE CONVENTIONAL AMERICAN DIET. ITS CAPACITY TO DISRUPT AND DEGRADE YOUR NATURAL

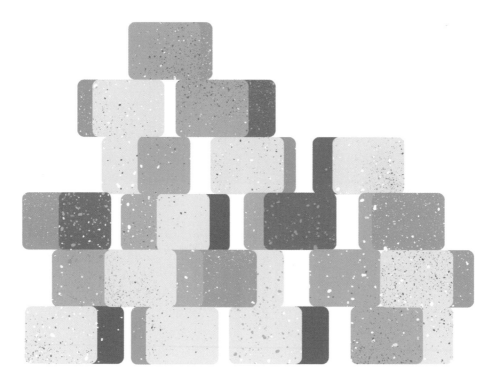

BALANCE IS NOTORIOUS. IT ALTERS YOUR HORmones so you don't register hunger the way you normally should, making you eat more. It spikes your dopamine, requiring you to eat more sugar to get that "sugar high" effect. Worst of all, when it's in the form of fructose, it affects your liver in the same way that alcohol does. Ingesting it consistently sets you up for inflammation and weight gain, leads to insulin resistance (the precursor to diabetes and heart disease), and lays the groundwork for every flavor of modern distress, from cancer, dementia, and depression, to infertility, acne,

and more. When combined with the underactive modern lifestyle, sugar changes your metabolic functioning—you go from a new sports car to an old, brokendown jalopy. To make matters worse, sugar also fuels candida—an unwanted fungus that can colonize the microbiome and throw it out of balance.

Given sugar's insidious presence in the modern food system and its highly addictive nature, you have to be on your game—and poised to push back. Sugar is everywhere, and nobody can say "no" to it but you.

WHO, ME?
I HARDLY EAT SUGAR!

Even if you don't eat sweets, you're likely ingesting more sugar than you think. Food manufacturers have managed to smuggle it into much (or most) of the modern food landscape. Of the almost 80,000 processed foods on the market, 58 percent of them contain added sugar—and not just to sweeten the taste! Sugar is a cheap preservative that extends food's shelf life while keeping you hooked.

Even people who eat clean tend to underestimate the total "free sugars" they consume in a day. "Free sugars" means any sugars added to a food, like table sugar or high-fructose corn syrup (which as a group is commonly called "added sugars"), *as well as any naturally occurring sugar in a food that is not bound by fiber, like fruit juice, honey, maple syrup, and agave.* (Free sugars do not include the naturally occurring sugars in milk, fruits, and vegetables, though these carbohydrates also turn to glucose in the blood to be used as energy; see Customize Your Carbs, page 85.) Seen through this lens, even healthy-seeming foods, like a post-workout protein bar or date-filled smoothie, can be quietly increasing your daily sugar tally. Liquid sugars are the worst: The fructose in juices and sweet beverages goes straight to the liver, where it is metabolized in a way similar to alcohol and converted into fat. Not only is this process a major driver of obesity, it damages the liver and can ultimately lead to fatty liver disease.

Start tallying all the ways you meet sugar in a day—from innocent-seeming foods like organic (but secretly sweetened) peanut butter or ketchup, or moments grabbing a snack or drink—and it can induce sugar shock. The small traces really do add up: Some researchers have deduced that the average American consumes 77 pounds of cane- and corn-derived sugars a year, much of it hard to detect because it's called by a bevy of other names in the ingredients you see on food labels (see Know the Codes, page 28).

Sugar is an extraordinarily destructive substance that most people eat far too much of.

FRUCTOSE IS NOT YOUR FRIEND

Glucose and fructose are the two "simple sugar" carbohydrates your body metabolizes, and together, they make sucrose (table sugar). For years, doctors, myself included, thought that fructose, the natural sugar in fruits and vegetables (which gets refined into things like the high-fructose corn syrup used in processed foods and drinks and is naturally occurring in agave syrup) was safe, as its impact on blood sugar levels is lower than that of glucose. We now know different: Fructose is metabolized by the liver and is not used by the brain or muscles for energy like glucose. High levels of fructose in the diet trigger fat production, increases in triglycerides, and, over time, fatty liver and hepatic insulin resistance. Fruit juices and anything sweetened by corn products will derail your efforts to stay well.

KNOW THE CODES

Sugars get sneaked into foods in a myriad of forms. Just a few of the key words you should look for include: cane sugar, brown sugar, brown rice syrup, beet sugar, date sugar, grape sugar, glucose, sucrose, maltose, maltodextrin, dextran, dextrose, sorbitol, corn syrup, fructose, high-fructose corn syrup, fructose syrup, corn sugar, fruit juice, fruit juice concentrate, barley malt, caramel, carob syrup, and sorghum syrup.

KICKING SUGAR TO THE CURB

Addicted to sugar and want to really break the cycle? Take the bull by the horns and commit to an elimination diet (page 90), because eliminating flour, baked goods, and even artificial sweeteners helps to powerfully reduce cravings for the sweeter stuff. When you eat a fiber-rich, whole-foods diet, the bacteria in your microbiome send messages to the brain that it's been well fed, helping to curb the cravings for a hit of sugar.

And be careful with alternative sugars: Coconut sugar—a new favorite of the health world—is still sugar, albeit with traces of more minerals. Raw honey, which has healing properties in small amounts, is also sugar, so tread carefully with your teaspoon. When needing a touch of sweet, try stevia, monk fruit, or xylitol, which are safer non-sugar options—but use them in moderation. The idea is to accustom your taste buds to foods that are less sweet, not more. And always avoid artificial sweeteners, which disrupt your microbiome, have neurotoxic properties, and trigger cravings, setting off a vicious cycle for those trying to avoid sweets.

To get the full lowdown on Big Sugar, and why life is so much sweeter without it, watch the documentary *Sugar Coated*.

RISE UP AND WISE UP

Though food labels list grams of sugar per serving, it's easier to picture the impact on your body when you convert this number to teaspoons. Four grams equals 1 teaspoon of sugar. On average we are consuming 22 teaspoons of added sugars a day in the form of sweetening agents in processed foods and sugar added to foods and drinks—and some people consume much more. Your bloodstream has only about 2 teaspoons of glucose (blood sugar) circulating in it to maintain equilibrium before you eat; anything else must be either burned or stored. (Since there is only so much glucose we need to burn in order to have energy, the overload gets stored, first as glycogen in your liver and muscles and then, when those storage tanks are full, all over your body as fat.) The mechanism for shunting the glucose out of the bloodstream and into cells and tissues is insulin, a hormone secreted by the pancreas. When insulin is constantly being released to handle continual inputs of glucose, the cells can stop responding to the insulin, and insulin levels then increase in the blood. This state is known as insulin resistance, and it is by far the most important risk factor for hypertension, heart disease, diabetes, and obesity (and probably Alzheimer's), not cholesterol levels as is commonly believed.

To keep things safely in check, avoid packaged foods and drinks that list a sugar content of over 4 grams per serving and don't use recipes that go above that, either. Also limit your intake of honey, maple syrup, coconut water, and fruit juice, foods that can trip you up even when following a clean and unprocessed whole-foods diet. You can also look at the ingredient list on food labels: If sugar or one of its sneakily worded siblings is one of the first three ingredients, back away. Doing this consistently will give you Sugar Survival Skills. And remember: Savory does not mean sugar-free.

Nixing the sugar from your coffee or cutting the ice cream habit are the hard-hitting ways to cut sugar. But to effectively lower your daily load, you also need to look for the small doses that accumulate in processed foods, condiments, and drinks grabbed on the run.

LOW-FAT FRUIT YOGURT: 6 to 12 cubes
KETCHUP: 1 cube
BBQ SAUCE: 3 to 4 cubes
BAKED BEANS: 5 cubes
VANILLA LATTE: 9 cubes
"AMERICAN" STYLE PEANUT BUTTER: 1 to 2 cubes
SWEETENED ICED TEA: 6 to 7 cubes
PICKLES: 2 cubes
GRANOLA: 3 to 6 cubes
BOTTLED FRUIT SMOOTHIE: 10 to 15 cubes
SPAGHETTI SAUCE: 5 cubes
SWEET DESSERT WINE: 5 cubes (dry white wine is just under 1 cube)
SPORTS DRINK: 8 to 9 cubes
ORANGE JUICE: 5 to 6 cubes
PROTEIN BAR: 5 to 6 cubes

*1 cube equals 1 teaspoon of sugar

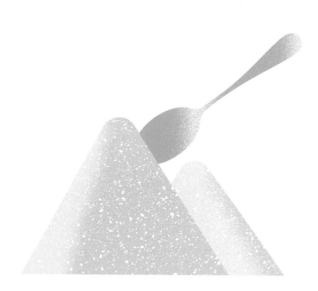

MAKE FRIENDS WITH FAT

IF YOUR DIET IS LEAN AND MEAN, PLEASE FATTEN IT UP. EATING A DIET OF LOW-FAT FOODS IS NOT THE TICKET TO HEALTH WE ONCE THOUGHT. FAT IS ABSOLUTELY ESSENTIAL FOR EVERY FUNCTION OF THE BODY AND BRAIN, INCLUDING HEALING AND REPAIRING FUNCTIONS, AND WHEN YOU EAT ENOUGH OF IT EVERY DAY, YOU ENJOY

A BOUNTY OF BENEFITS: STABLE, LONGER-LASTING energy and fewer hunger highs and lows; a more efficient metabolism (meaning more stable weight); clearer thinking and more balanced moods; healthier hormones; better hair, nails, and skin; and fewer cravings. And because fat makes food taste good, you enjoy what you're eating so much more.

Plenty has been written about *why* fatty foods were so wrongly demonized for the last five decades (my favorite sources: Nina Teicholz's book, *The Big Fat Surprise*, and Dr. Aseem Malhotra's excellent book, *The Pioppi Diet*). Our culture bought into this demonization—diligently following government guidelines and Big Food's marketing—and it led to a dangerous and damaging tidal wave of carbohydrates, refined sugars, seed oils, and fake foods coursing through our modern food system. Now we're waking up to new insights about fat's central role in health, such as the realization that women are at a higher risk of heart attack on a low-fat diet than a high-fat one, and the importance of cholesterol to the body's functions (see page 251). It's time to repair the relationship, steering it back onto its natural track.

If the thought of eating more fat sends shivers down your spine, do not fear. This initiative is about adding real-food fats to your plate—naturally fat-rich foods and unprocessed fats in their original states—and letting them crowd out the refined carbs and sugar that might otherwise take up the space. Real-food fats not only deliver powerful protective benefits, they are hard to overeat because they digest more slowly, giving your brain and hunger-regulating hormones more time to register fullness.

You don't need a rigorous dietary plan to accomplish this. Just focus on adding fat-rich ingredients in small ways throughout the day while simultaneously being careful to keep your starches and sugars *low*, because adding extra fats to a high-carbohydrate diet will certainly encourage weight gain. Keep it simple, keep it consistent, and soon you will forge a fast—and enduring—friendship with this super-powered macronutrient.

HOW TO FATIFY YOUR DIET

The complicated lingo around fats can get confusing (saturated, poly-, mono-, and omegas). My general rule of thumb for fat: If it comes from nature, it's probably healthy, and if it's made in a factory, be it feedlot or processing plant, it's probably not. (In other words, blocks of orange cheese or potato chips are not the way to go.) And be cautious: Even with healthy fats, high fat plus excessive carbohydrates will derail you. In other words, pick the unsweetened coconut yogurt—or the grass-fed, whole-milk kind—over the gourmet, but sugary, ice cream. The rigorous research trials that show the success of higher-fat diets at countering obesity, diabetes, and heart disease (such as ketogenic diets, page 84) all follow *high-fat, low-carbohydrate* protocols.

The subject becomes simple if you think about the following three categories that correspond with the ways we eat fat-rich foods. Integrate them into your routine from morning to night, using the general ratios described in Compose the Perfect Plate (page 23), as a guide. This is about consuming small amounts—it doesn't mean that every meal should be dripping with oils or laden with strips of bacon! How to know if you're getting enough fat? Your body will give you the cues: Pay attention to your energy level, feeling of satiety, and the resolution of any symptoms of fat deficit, such as brittle hair and nails.

»

Fat-free living has had the opposite effect on our health; instead of making us healthier, we have obesity and diabetes epidemics.

«

FAT-RICH FOODS

The raw materials you use as part of your meals and snacks. Be careful about your sources—the fattier the food, the more important that it comes from a quality source, as nutrient value *and* toxins accumulate in fat. (Be sure to read the Clean Eating Cheat Sheet on page 147.)

ANIMAL FOODS

ORGANIC CHICKEN WITH SKIN (DARK MEAT)
GRASS-FED AND -FINISHED RED MEAT
(some cuts are lean, others are fattier; ask your butcher)
PASTURED PORK, INCLUDING PORK BELLY AND BACON
LAMB
EGGS, IDEALLY PASTURE-RAISED AND ORGANIC
FATTY COLD-WATER FISH
(sardines, mackerel, herring, wild salmon)
DAIRY THAT WORKS FOR YOU
(goat and sheep cheese; cow cheese if tolerated; grass-fed butter; yogurt/kefir)
BONE BROTHS

PLANT FOODS

AVOCADO
COCONUT
(oil, butter, milk, cream)
NUTS AND NUT BUTTERS
(in moderation; preferably raw [unroasted])
SEEDS
(pumpkin, chia, sesame, flax, hemp)
CHOCOLATE (see page 64)
OLIVES AND OLIVE OIL

POURING AND SPREADING FATS

The things you drizzle, spread, or spoon over your food (or into your smoothie or coffee) straight from the bottle: olive oil, flax oil, hemp oil, nut oils, nut butters, MCT oil (liquid coconut), cacao butter, dairy butter, and ghee.

COOKING FATS

What you use to make raw food cooked! Animal fats like ghee and butter, duck fat, pork fat, chicken fat, tallow (to sear your protein); plant oils like coconut oil, sustainably sourced palm oil, avocado oil, and quality olive oils. Turn to page 76 for a guide to safe pouring and cooking fats.

A DAY WITH MORE FAT: IDEAS FOR MORNING TO NIGHT

NOURISHING SMOOTHIE
(see page 67) with added nut butter, MCT oil, or chunks of frozen avocado
FAT-ENHANCED (AKA BULLETPROOF) COFFEE with added MCT oil, grass-fed butter, or grass-fed cream
EGGS COOKED IN GHEE OR BUTTER
SARDINES WITH AVOCADO
SLOW-COOKED PORK OR LAMB STEW
on vegetables or salad
EVOO DRIZZLED OVER VEGETABLES AND PROTEINS
BONE BROTH
for sustenance throughout the day
TAHINI SAUCE
drizzled over a vegetable and rice bowl
ALMOND BUTTER DRESSING
for zucchini noodles
BRUSSELS SPROUTS WITH BACON
DARK CHOCOLATE
COCONUT MILK CURRY
COCONUT YOGURT CHIA PUDDING
(or dairy yogurt if tolerated)
A SPOONFUL OF GHEE IN YOUR EVENING TEA

9 (MORE) REASONS TO EMBRACE NATURAL FATS

THEY HELP your body absorb critical vitamins (the fat-soluble vitamins A, D, E, and K).
THEY STRENGTHEN your immune system.
THEY SUPPORT proper integrity of your cell membranes.
THEY FEED the unique needs of your brain.
THEY LUBRICATE your digestive system.
THEY PROTECT your vital organs.
THEY HELP reduce inflammation.
THEY FEED your mitochondria, the cellular powerhouses that determine how energized you feel and how you age.
THEY ARE essential for the health of your heart, lungs, liver, and bones and help healthy gene expression.

My general rule of thumb for fat: If it comes from nature, it's probably healthy, and if it's made in a factory, be it feedlot or processing plant, it's probably not.

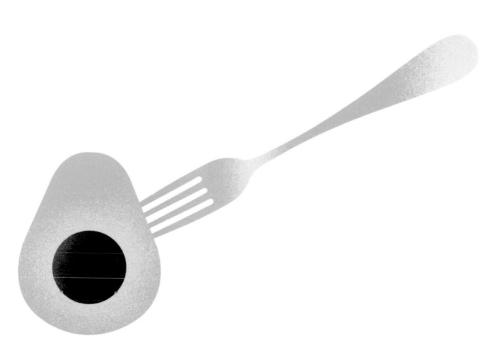

HOW TO GO **GLUTEN-FREE**

OF ALL THE DIETARY INTERVENTIONS I SUGGEST TO PATIENTS WHO DON'T FEEL WELL, CUTTING OUT GLUTEN TENDS TO DELIVER SOME OF THE MOST RAPIDLY DETECTABLE RESULTS. WHEN WHEAT AND OTHER GLUTEN-CONTAINING PRODUCTS ARE TAKEN OFF THE PLATE OF SOMEONE WHO IS SENSITIVE TO THEM, DIGESTIVE

ISSUES CAN LESSEN; ENERGY AND MENTAL CLARITY return; persistent aches, pains, and stiffness dissolve; and headaches can subside—and that's just a sampling. The bumper-sticker motto in these cases? *I didn't realize I was feeling so crummy until I didn't feel so crummy.* In some more serious cases, this one new habit is the crucial first step to turning around a serious autoimmune condition.

But how do you know if *you* should steer clear of this plant-based protein, which is found in wheat and other grains like rye and barley; wheat's many relatives like wheat germ, bulgur, couscous, farina, semolina, and spelt; and a smorgasbord of processed foods and drinks that smuggle this protein into their mixes without you even realizing? And, if you decide to do it, how do you chart a safe and steady course through gluten-free's glittering ocean of fancy processed products and far-out promises? Welcome to Gluten-Free 2.0—it's time to learn how to go against the grain in a way that heals but won't hurt.

WHEAT'S BAD RAP

Although wheat has been known as the "staff of life" for over eight thousand years, I believe that our off-balance microbiomes, with the inflamed intestines that result, might be triggering increasing intolerance. The sheer amount of wheat we consume (it comprises at least 20 percent of the average Westerner's daily diet) may be partly to blame, and the industrialized processes behind modern wheat, which is the largest global food crop, seem to present clear-and-present dangers. Today's high-speed baking technologies sidestep traditional techniques that helped break down the protein into more digestible sizes. Worse is the alarming use of the herbicide glyphosate in conventional wheat production (see page 153).

When you are sensitive to gluten, the inflammation that results can manifest anywhere in the body. It can cause digestive distress, headaches, achy joints, all kinds of

Lifestyle factors, especially diet, heavily influence what roughly 98 percent of our genes do, how they behave, and how they express themselves.

neurological issues, bloating, skin imbalances, ovarian cysts, and more. (It can also be the cause of the autoimmune syndrome celiac disease, which creates disturbance body-wide, as well as contribute to a host of other autoimmune syndromes.)

The good news is that removing gluten-containing foods, and then improving microbiome health, typically resolves many of the chronic inflammatory symptoms. It can even restore a level of functioning that allows some sensitive folk to enjoy occasional portions of well-prepared gluten foods. (If you have celiac disease, in which the delicate microvilli in your intestines get damaged, this will not be the case, but removing gluten religiously will allow the villi to heal.)

There's another reason to consider reducing your gluten dependence. Bread in particular is a notorious blood-sugar destabilizer. Cutting it out can help you lose weight.

STOP! DROP THAT GLUTEN-FREE MUFFIN!

The first wave of gluten-free eating launched an entire industry of processed and packaged foods, many of which are riddled with high-carbohydrate starches and industrial seed oils, not to mention sugar, preservatives, and additives. Ignore most of them. They invite high blood sugar, inflammation, and weight gain. To make this transition healthfully, *follow the tips in this book*. Eat real food. Eschew packaged foods. Let vegetables crowd out the pasta or bread and practice composing the Perfect Plate (page 23). Gluten-free products can help in a pinch—and there are some great ones out there that are devoid of seed oils and additives—but don't make them a crutch. Then this dietary change can kick-start a long-lasting and sustainable way of eating.

GOING GLUTEN-FREE VERSION 2.0

Do you do better with cold-turkey quitting or slowly tapering off? To go gluten-free, pick the path that suits you, follow the guidelines, and use the Food Sensitivities Questionnaire from howtobewell.com to help you chart any changes in your symptoms. (If you're wondering about blood tests for gluten sensitivities, read the box on page 91.)

Whichever pathway you choose, stay on it for at least two weeks. Take note of any shifts in how you feel and look. If you have been suffering from symptoms for some time, the real work of healing an inflamed gut wall, and possibly assisting in the resolution of any autoimmune conditions, is a several-months-long process. Keep on it!

PATHWAY 1: START WITH BREAKFAST

An incremental phasing-out that lets you gain your footing one step at a time. If you are not in a crisis of uncomfortable symptoms, or if you are overwhelmed by huge changes or by the idea of throwing out food from your pantry, this method can work well. Typically, even only changing breakfast helps you regain energy and feel better, and it delivers a surge of enthusiasm to take the next step. As you tackle each meal, get rid of the gluten-containing products in your kitchen that supply it.

HOW TO DO IT:
Start by replacing any gluten foods at your morning meal. Remember, savory leftovers can be a great breakfast. Note: If you're eating oatmeal, make sure it is gluten-free (oats are technically not a gluten grain, but are often cross-contaminated due to the shared machinery used in harvesting and milling).

Commit to this one act for one week. Notice any changes in how you are feeling.

The following week, replace the gluten foods at lunch. Commit to this for one week, and keep noticing how you feel.

Now that you have breakfast and lunch handled, on week three, change dinner. Look carefully at your snack choices, too.

Make sure to think in advance about eating out, and have

a strategy for where you will eat and what you will order (see page 74).

PATHWAY 2: THE CLEAN SWEEP

The cold-turkey method. This method works well if you are highly motivated, either because you are sick of suffering or you do better when you are accountable to stricter goals.

HOW TO DO IT:

Before you start, take a few days to plan how you will eat, ideally writing out a strategy and making several lists. Review the entire How to Eat section of this book. Consider: What will I eat for three meals a day, plus snacks? What do I need to throw out of my kitchen and workplace? What will I replace this with? What will I do when I eat out? What will I do if I slip?

The Clean Sweep can be part of a broader elimination diet (page 90) or, better yet, part of a full gut repair program (page 174) if you are ready to go the whole hog of rebooting your digestion, calming inflammation, and restoring the microbiome.

SUCCEEDING IN THE SHIFT

UNMASK AND AVOID HIDDEN SOURCES OF GLUTEN, such as the thickeners and fillers in processed foods, sauces, some sausages, and desserts. (A quick internet search will deliver you comprehensive lists.)

SUBSTITUTE WISELY. Use the content in this ring to help you come up with wheat-free meals and snacks, and consult the plethora of websites devoted to gluten-free cooking for even more ideas. When in doubt, just eat more vegetables!

BE OKAY WITH NOT FEELING OKAY. Gluten has an opioid effect: When you consume it, your body actually makes a hormone—a gluten endorphin—that raises your mood. No wonder it's so addictive! Cutting it out can feel like drug withdrawal at first. If cravings for your former gluten foods kick in, eat some quality protein and good fats to satiate yourself wisely.

IF YOU FALL OFF THE WAGON, DON'T STRESS. Notice if any symptoms arise immediately after you eat gluten foods, or the next morning. These might include fatigue, foggy head, aches, pains, digestive issues, and constipation. Let them be your signposts to get you back on track.

SEIZE THIS EXCITING OPPORTUNITY TO MAKE NEW FOODS! Paleo bread sounds intimidating until you see how short the ingredient list is. There have never been more resources, blogs, and good ingredients available to those who want to cook gluten-free. Don't try to wing it without healthy food and snacks on hand. You will get hungry and desperate!

AFTER TWO WEEKS

Assess the impact of this shift by reviewing the Food Sensitivities Questionnaire again. How do you feel without gluten-containing foods, compared to before you cut them from your diet? What happens now when you eat a piece of bread or some pasta? You might find that the

Of all the interventions I suggest to patients who don't feel well, cutting out gluten tends to deliver some of the most rapidly detectable results.

LECTINS: LOOKING *BEYOND* GLUTEN

If removing gluten from your diet does not resolve symptoms caused by inflammation and leaky gut, it might be wise to learn about lectins, the larger family of plant proteins of which gluten is a member. Lectins are proteins found in many plants (especially beans and legumes, including peanuts) as well as in grains and the seeds and peels of nightshades. These proteins evolved as part of the plant's survival strategy, deliberately causing discomfort or distress in predators' bodies so that they would not be eaten and could then reproduce. Some people are sensitive to these proteins and experience instant digestive distress or inflammation. Others coexist with them tolerably, especially when foods containing lectins are properly cooked, because lectin content is dramatically reduced by traditional cooking methods such as soaking, sprouting, fermenting, and even refining beans, legumes, and grains. These traditional methods, as well as the uncompromised quality of preindustrial ingredients and the abundance of helpful pre- and probiotic foods in the diet, helped make grains and beans successful staples of many global cultures.

If you are sensitive to lectins, these preparation methods may be your key to happily enjoying the plant foods that contain them, and they are easy to learn. For example, pressure cooking is a great way to reduce lectin content, particularly in beans or legumes, so consider learning how to use this high-speed and very helpful kitchen technique (page 53).

If you are trying to resolve stubborn food sensitivities, you may want to cut all lectin-containing foods from your diet and then reintroduce them one by one to see which you are sensitive to. Dairy, factory-farmed meats, and eggs even contain lectins, which may be why a true elimination diet that cuts these out resolves issues for some sensitive people.)

For a deep dive into the subject of lectins, read The Plant Paradox *by Steven R. Gundry, MD.*

results are intolerable. You might find they are moderate, making it okay to occasionally include these foods in your diet, as a conscious choice. Or you might find that eating that bread or pasta doesn't seem to affect you at all. Whatever the result, you have kick-started a *gluten-aware* way of eating, something I believe to be an invaluable key to being well in a world where our food sources, and our bodies' responses to them, are undeniably changing.

AFTER THREE MONTHS

If your gut was inflamed by gluten, you may find this time off has allowed some healing to occur. You may be able to tolerate small amounts of authentic sourdough bread, which is fermented and therefore easier to digest (see page 56). Sprouted wheat products may also be easier to digest (see page 37), though I would *always* suggest you eat some spinach or chard in place of any kind of bread or baked goods, and zucchini or summer squash ribbons in place of pasta. But no matter what, try to ensure that any wheat or grain you buy is organic, especially if you are feeding it to your kids!

To get the full picture on gluten, check out the movie *What's With Wheat?* and the books *Grain Brain* by David Perlmutter, MD, and *Wheat Belly* by William Davis, MD.

RESIST THE IRRESISTIBLE:
PROCESSED FOODS

YOU'VE HEARD IT A HUNDRED TIMES: HIGHLY PROCESSED JUNK FOODS, FAST FOODS, AND SODAS WILL HURT YOU BADLY. FOOD IS INFORMATION THAT TELLS YOUR ENTIRE BIOLOGY WHAT TO DO AND WHEN TO DO IT, BUT JUNK FOOD IS LIKE MALWARE ON YOUR COMPUTER: SCRAMBLED INFORMATION THAT LEADS TO A MAJOR

HARDWARE CRASH. FOOD MADE BY AN INDUSTRIAL, manmade manufacturing system is many steps away from what nature intended, and the sneaky cocktail of seed oils, hidden sugars, GMOs, chemical colorants, texturizers, and preservatives used to make processed and junk foods so palatable—and so cheap—disrupt all of the Four Directions outlined on page 14. They do this by triggering inflammation that leads to weight gain, brain fog, and system-wide pain (often doing damage silently and unnoticed for years); disrupting the balance of hormones (such as through estrogenic chemicals); degrading your microbiome and possibly contributing to food allergies; and, because they are so highly engineered to be addictive, disrupting your natural rhythms of eating (i.e., regularly consuming simple, whole foods and finding them fully satiating).

Breaking free of the grip of processed food is a must if you want to claim and own your health. If boxed, packaged, and logo-covered food is a big part of your diet, it's going to take some revolutionary tactics to fuel a successful resistance, but it's worth it: weight loss, digestive ease, mental clarity, better skin, better sleep, and more stable moods are the prize that you win. Here are my best tactics for breaking free.

1. GET ANGRY: YOU'VE BEEN HIJACKED!

Convenience foods are convenient only for the companies that profit off them. Junk food and fast food have been engineered by food scientists to be *hyper-palatable*, which means they will put anything in them to make you crave their taste and texture. Typically that includes high doses

of sugar, bad oils, MSG, GMO soy, and chemical flavorings (the "artificial flavor" listed can contain countless unnamed chemicals). A hyper-palatable food is designed to derail your satiety signaling; it will induce cravings to overeat, trigger an unnatural food high via a dopamine reaction in your body, and override your innate ability to stop eating (hence the infamous marketing lines like "Once you pop, you just can't stop!"). This unregulated food engineering adds up to one big science experiment that doesn't work in your favor, but it sure makes money for shareholders. Remember this: Many processed foods, most fast food, and almost every soda in the world have been *designed and built* with addiction in mind. (This includes the fare at many fast casual restaurants that tempt you with "handcrafted" onion rings or "authentic" cheesy-floury-meaty burritos. A recent survey found 83 percent of Americans eat out because of cravings.)

To get the lowdown on shady Big Food practices, check out the book *Salt, Sugar, Fat: How the Food Giants Hooked Us* by Michael Moss.

2. LEARN TO SPEED READ

If your food's ingredient list exceeds three to five ingredients, be on alert.

If you can't pronounce or easily identify the ingredients (no matter how few or many there are), that's red flag number one.

Don't let the front of the bag seduce you. Even "organic, stone-ground corn chips" are likely made with inflammatory seed oils. And many processed foods use refined palm oil or "vegetable oils"; they're highly inflammatory, too. Turn the product over and take a closer look.

Avoid "low-fat" and "sugar-free" products. To compensate for what's missing, nefarious ingredients like fake sweeteners are added, which can induce even more cravings.

If sugars are over 4g per serving, evaluate carefully, and if you see high-fructose corn syrup listed, stop immediately—game over.

To cut to the chase, try scanning barcodes with an app like FoodFacts, which gives a snapshot of all the hidden nasties and allergens lurking in an item, or read the guide *Chemical Cuisine,* from the Center for Science in the Public Interest (cspinet.org), which decodes the additives listed.

Additionally, my health coaches swear by the Healthy Living app from the Environmental Working Group, which scores a huge database of foods.

3. STRUCTURE YOUR EATING

Getting in a rhythm of regularly timed meals provides a solid foundation so you are less vulnerable to junk food urges. Have reliable, healthy snacks on hand, drink plenty of water, and keep preprepared meal components in the fridge. Be sure to get enough well-sourced protein, healthy fat, and fiber from vegetables in your diet. These are the bedrock actions supporting toxin-free eating.

4. KNOW YOUR FOOD TRIGGERS

Practice "inserting a pause" when the urge for a junk-food fix arises. Take a breath. Go for a walk. Notice what is happening in your body and mind when the desire hits. Typically, the trigger is boredom (wanting a change of activity), fatigue (needing energy), or sorrow/loneliness (wanting comfort). Increasing your awareness of *why* you want what you want gives you the tools to resist the craving and make an empowered, better choice. There are numerous books and online resources related to mindful and intuitive eating to help you on this path—support is only a click away.

Breaking free of the grip of processed food is a must if you want to claim and own your health.

KNOW YOUR SOURCES

THOUGH AMERICANS HAVE LONG BEEN OBSESSED WITH *QUANTITY* OF FOOD AS IT RELATES TO HEALTH AND WEIGHT, IT'S THE *QUALITY* OF THE FOOD THAT MATTERS MOST. TOXIN-FREE FOODS THAT ARE NUTRITIOUS THE WAY NATURE INTENDED (MINIMALLY PROCESSED) GIVE YOUR BODY THE RIGHT SIGNALS TO STAY IN BALANCE.

BUT WITH OUR DEEPLY FLAWED FOOD SYSTEM, IT takes commitment to source and buy quality food—depending on where you live, it can feel like a battle. It's crazy that it should be that way, but there's the rub: We have an industrial food supply that has favored profit over health for so long that it's made disease-causing foods mainstream and health-giving foods fringe.

Luckily, we're riding a big wave of change. Millions of people are demanding a shift from industrial food to integrity food: nutrition that is affordable, accessible, and bursting with fresh and healthful properties. Thanks to consumer demand, there are more farmers' markets, manufacturers are changing harmful processes, and we *are* slowly cleaning up the mess. But the momentum will only continue to build if we all engage! Here are five ways to be part of the shift and see your (and your family's) health skyrocket as a result.

1. KEEP IT SIMPLE.

Stick mainly to unfussy meals made of whole foods. Find what you like and use it often. If you commit to cooking and dial back on eating out, you'll have some extra cash to spend on quality where it costs more, such as healthfully raised meat, dairy, eggs, and fish.

2. KNOW THE SOURCE OF YOUR FOOD.

The good food providers *want* you to be engaged. They are transparent about their processes and willing to share. Meet the farmers at your local farmers' market. Ask questions. Support their hard work. Consider joining a CSA (community-supported agriculture) project to secure a season of fresh food (see localharvest.com). Same goes for brands you buy: Read their websites, share your concerns, leave your comments on the sites you buy from. Brands with integrity listen.

3. BE A MARKETING SKEPTIC.

The food business is notoriously slippery, and marketing lingo is artfully selected not only to get you to buy on impulse without thinking but also to give a product a "health halo"—an identity that projects an aura of wellness without the reality. Be wary of hyped-up phrases that don't tell you anything! The word "natural" is unregulated except for meat and poultry, where it means only that no additives or processing occurred; "natural" can even be splashed on a product that is made with genetically engineered ingredients. "Contains whole grains" tells you nothing useful for your health, and "farm fresh" is equally empty—factory farms are farms, too, after all. Read the fine print and do your research on the products you use frequently.

4. VOTE WITH YOUR DOLLAR.

Organic is no longer the alternative option as the market for it expands at a rapid pace. Make your purchases chemical-free as much as you can (see page 147). Get vocal and buy local. It's still an uphill battle for people who are making and growing food the right way! We continue to subsidize the mono crops and factory-farmed animal foods that inflame us and make us fat, while small, local producers supplying organic, whole foods get no help. The more you support those devoted to quality products, buy from alternative retailers like thrivemarket.com (which is 100 percent GMO-free), or take a personal step like growing your own produce in a community garden or sprouting on your kitchen counter (page 170), the more you help build an alternative food system.

Another good reason to spring for organic: The more you buy it, the more you help our degraded soils get healthier. The soil has a microbiome just like you do, a thriving world of biota that ensures its robust good health. But that's been decimated by years of chemical-based and genetically engineered agriculture, which means it can't feed plants the high levels of nutrients that it should. Buying organic helps repair this injustice, and the better the health of the soil, the better the health of the food, and that ripples out to you.

5. STAY VIGILANT.

The playing field is constantly shifting. Big corporations are buying up the organic market and taking over small real-food companies. Dilution of quality and subtle shifts (like adding cheaper but toxic ingredients or downgrading original sources) can occur. Also, regulations on dangerous chemicals are not safeguarded—the food industry generally gets to declare what is safe and what's not, operating fully on their own terms—and frighteningly, long-standing bans on some dangerous pesticides, like the carcinogen chlorpyrifos, are being overturned. The regulatory system is broken, and it is no secret that special-interest money speaks louder than consumer safety. Don't fall asleep at the wheel—fixing this broken food system requires participation and more than a little vigilance! Luckily, there are dedicated groups doing most of the hard work for you. Use their resources, support their initiatives (such as pushing for the labeling of genetically engineered foods), and become part of the solution. For more information, visit the websites of my favorite integrity leaders in the area of food quality and safety:

- **ENVIRONMENTAL WORKING GROUP:** ewg.org

- **FOOD DEMOCRACY NOW:** fooddemocracynow.org

- **ORGANIC CONSUMERS ASSOCIATION:** organicconsumers.org

- **THE CORNUCOPIA INSTITUTE:** cornucopia.org

- **PESTICIDE ACTION NETWORK:** panna.org

- **CENTER FOR FOOD SAFETY:** centerforfoodsafety.org

We have an industrial food supply that has favored profit over health for so long that it's made disease-causing foods mainstream and health-giving foods fringe.

>>

The emerging science of epigenetics is revealing how the environment around you and your lifestyle choices play a huge role in whether you get sick or stay healthy.

<<

DOCTOR UP YOUR BROTH

IN TRADITIONAL CUISINES AROUND THE GLOBE, IT IS A COMMON DAILY PRACTICE TO SERVE BROTH MADE FROM MEAT, FISH, OR VEGETABLES. I PROPOSE WE DO THE SAME. IN MY PRACTICE I FREQUENTLY PRESCRIBE BROTH AS PART OF A PROTOCOL FOR HEALING THE GUT—AND AS A FORTIFYING, HEALTH-PROMOTING

TONIC THAT FITS INTO A TIME-PRESSED LIFE. HAVE you noticed that humble bone broth has earned "souper-food" status today? The reasons are many: Not only is collagen (broth's easily absorbable protein structure) gently and quickly nourishing, it is healing and supportive for taxed and damaged digestive systems. Broth delivers important good fats, fat-soluble vitamins, and minerals; counters inflammation and supports the joints and skin; and boosts your immune system (hot broth in winter – obvious preventive tool). And when you have broth in your kitchen, you have a nutrition-rich base for easy-to-make soups and stews.

Two things can help you make broth-drinking a daily habit: Have it on hand in your kitchen, ready to heat (see page 44 for a recipe, or order frozen broth from quality sources like brodobroth.myshopify.com or bonafidepro-visions.com). And find the way you like it best: plain and simple, or spiked with a shake or splash of flavor. Start by sipping broth before a meaty meal (it helps the digestive system break down the proteins) or as a warming cup when you would otherwise grab a tea. It can give a satisfying lift first thing in the morning—a broth spiked with coconut oil or ghee might tempt you to skip coffee entirely—or a light end to the day, letting your digestion rest before you go to bed.

SPIKE IT, FROTH IT: INSIDER SECRETS FROM MARCO CANORA

Chef **Marco Canora** is not only a longtime client and friend, he's the Broth Guru: author of *Brodo*, a bone broth cookbook, founder of Brodo broth bar in New York, and famed for bringing irresistible and unexpected hot-broth drinks into fashion (one of his specialties is *tom yum* brodo: chicken broth + chili oil + coconut milk + lime + curry spice blend). By grating turmeric or pouring ginger juice straight into the cup, or building depth by adding shiitake tea (water from soaking dry shiitake mushrooms) or garlic puree, Marco has helped harried New Yorkers discover that broth can be a great vehicle for flavor. Borrow his best tips and discover this for yourself.

HOW TO BE WELL EXPERT

3 TOOLS FOR DOCTORING YOUR BROTH

1. **A MORTAR AND PESTLE** for pounding fresh herbs or roots into a paste. Place the paste on the bottom of a cup and pour the hot broth over. The heat blossoms the flavor into your broth in a magical way.

2. **A BATTERY-OPERATED MILK FROTHER** for adding quality fats to your broth, like bone marrow, tallow, grass-fed ghee or butter, MCT oil, coconut oil, chili oil, or spicy EVOO. Blend dried spices or spice blends into the fat before you incorporate it into the broth to make a filling, delicious drink.

3. **A MICROPLANE** to grate literally anything into your broth. It's great for fresh ginger, turmeric, and garlic, but get creative and try some spicy radish or fresh horseradish.

HOW TO MAKE BONE BROTH

STEP 1: GATHER YOUR MATERIALS

You'll need 2 to 4 pounds of bones. They can be from poultry, fish, shellfish, beef, or lamb (look for 100 percent grass-fed or certified pastured meat). If using beef, try to include some meaty neck bones for maximum flavor. Another option: Use the carcass of a whole roast chicken, with any leftover meat on it. For this, you can use a smaller pot.

YOU WILL ALSO NEED:

- 1 gallon water, or enough to cover the bones by a few inches
- 3 to 4 tablespoons apple cider vinegar (or other natural vinegar) to draw out the minerals from the bones
- Large (8- to 12-quart) pot or slow cooker
- Mesh strainer or cheesecloth

Optional: vegetables (carrots, garlic, onion), sea salt, and herbs improve the flavor and can be added toward the end of the cooking time, if desired

STEP 2: FILL YOUR POT

Place the bones in your pot to fill it at least halfway; cover with water to within 1 inch from the top. Add vinegar and let sit for 30 to 60 minutes. Bring to a boil, then turn down to a simmer.

STEP 3: COOK AND WAIT

While it simmers, you can use a spoon to skim off any scum that rises to the top. Reduce the heat, cover, and allow the broth to simmer very gently. Cook on low heat for at least 6 hours or overnight, to extract the most gelatin and nutrients from the bones. A few hours before it is done, throw in the vegetables, sea salt, and herbs, if you are using them.

STEP 4: SEPARATE AND STORE

Remove from the heat and let cool. Pick out the heavy bones and discard, then strain the broth through a fine-mesh sieve or cheesecloth-lined strainer set over another pot or large bowl. When the broth is cool, ladle it into glass mason jars. The solid fat can stay on top of the broth until you are ready to use it; discard the fat before pouring. If you intend to freeze the broth, leave 2 inches of space at the top of the containers to allow for expansion, or freeze it without lids and then put the lids on after. Another option is to use freezer bags.

STEP 5: REHEAT AND SIP

When your broth is cooled, it should wiggle like jelly due to the high gelatin content (the cooked form of collagen)—that's the indication of a nourishing broth. Don't worry: When you warm it up in a pan, it will liquefy. If it doesn't turn gelatinous, it's still very good for you—just add more gristle into your mix next time (ask your butcher or provider for feet or knuckle bones, or add the skin from your roast chicken, and if you're making fish stock, be sure to include the nourishing head).

Your broth will keep for about 5 days in the fridge or 6 months in the freezer.

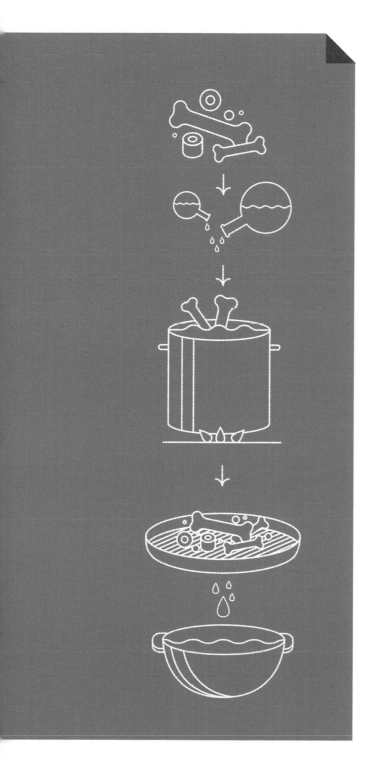

THE FLAVOR COMBOS

Play with ingredients and get to know their tastes. You don't need to be exact with the amounts. Add dashes and pinches of the following ingredients—start small and get to know the intensity of flavor you like.

- Seaweed (kelp, dulse, or noi) + ginger
- Coconut milk + ginger*
- Garlic puree + thyme or rosemary butter
- Shot of Bragg Liquid Aminos + whisk in an egg yolk
- Kimchi brine
- Parsley + fresh lemon juice
- Ras el hanout spice blend + butter + pulverized cilantro + squeeze of lime juice
- Garlic and dried or powdered mushrooms like shiitake, maitake, cordyceps, or reishi (this is an immunity-boosting drink)
- Ginger + fresh or ground turmeric (this is an anti-inflammatory drink)
- Coconut milk (one part milk to four parts broth) + pinch of ground turmeric + pinch of ground ginger + smashed garlic + pepper + salt*
- Cacao + coconut milk + cinnamon + coconut oil + maple syrup*

*best made using chicken broth, not beef

Quick substitute: Adding 1 to 2 tablespoons of powdered collagen to a simple vegetable broth can give you a healing and nourishing drink if you don't have bone broth on hand.

ANIMAL, VEGETABLE, MINERAL: WHAT IF I DON'T EAT MEAT?

Use leftover and wilting vegetables to make a mineral-rich vegetable broth. It won't have the same amino acid profile, but it's still considered a health tonic. And if you add seaweed (like kelp strips) or mushrooms (especially immune-boosting shiitake), you'll boost the mineral content further and get other medicinal qualities. Some vegetarians in need of gut help decide to use chicken, fish, or beef broth as part of their healing protocol.

DAIRY DO
OR DAIRY DON'T?

IS DAIRY THE DEVIL, AS SOME DAIRY-FREE ADVOCATES MIGHT HAVE YOU BELIEVE? IT'S MORE NUANCED THAN THAT. CLINICALLY, I'VE OBSERVED THAT DAIRY WORKS WELL FOR MANY PEOPLE, IRRITATES OTHERS, AND DOES VIOLENCE TO A FEW. SO WHEN IT COMES TO FIGURING OUT YOUR OWN RELATIONSHIP WITH THE STUFF, I DON'T

THINK IT'S THAT, WELL, BLACK OR WHITE. DON'T ASSUME you *have* to go cold turkey on all things milk-related, but on the quest for good health, determining what works for you, then committing to quality if you eat it, is a necessary project.

WHAT'S THE ISSUE?

Nixing dairy does often help clear up chronic symptoms like acne and other skin problems; digestive issues like constipation, diarrhea, acid reflux, and heartburn; and excessive mucus, congestion, and sinus irritation (not to mention weight gain—dairy is relatively high in carbohydrates). Usually these symptoms are caused by a sensitivity to the milk protein (normally the casein or, much less frequently, the whey), which triggers an inflammatory response. Digestive distress in particular might be caused by a deficiency in lactase, the enzymes required to break down milk sugars smoothly. Dairy intolerance often goes hand in hand with gluten intolerance, and it can be a contributor to autoimmune conditions; in those cases, nixing dairy can help tame the gut and cool inflammation.

BE A DAIRY DETECTIVE

If you experience any of those symptoms (or notice anything else unusual after eating dairy), it's a clue to do some digging. Follow the Food Sensitivity protocol on page 90. When the two weeks are over, see if you find profound relief from your symptoms. You do? Then you may want to steer clear of this food entirely (and make your own nut or seed milks, page 50).

However, it's not necessarily game-over. If going completely dairy-free feels too restrictive, try some personal exploration. In the reintroduction phase of the protocol, test the following foods one by one—they're the ones that can often be tolerated by people with mild cow's milk sensitivities. Note if they affect you or not.

1. **YOGURT AND/OR KEFIR** (unsweetened, with live active cultures). Fermented dairy is said to decrease lactose to less than 1 percent, rendering it much more digestible.

2. **GOAT- AND/OR SHEEP-MILK PRODUCTS.** These frequently work for people who are sensitive to cow's milk, though not always.

3. **HARD CHEESES** like Parmesan, pecorino, and other aged cheeses. These can be easier for those with lactose sensitivity because they are lower in the lactase sugars. This doesn't help if you are sensitive to the proteins found in cheese.

4. **GHEE (AKA CLARIFIED BUTTER).** Considered a healing food in India, partly because it contains gut-soothing butyric acid, ghee is butter oil without the milk protein, and it can be used for cooking and spreading. Look for ghee that has been verified to have almost no milk proteins.

5. **RAW MILK PRODUCTS.** Though there's no scientific consensus, anecdotal reports by users suggest raw dairy is often a "go" when pasteurized dairy is a "no," possibly because the enzymes needed to digest the proteins and sugars are still intact. If you can get raw

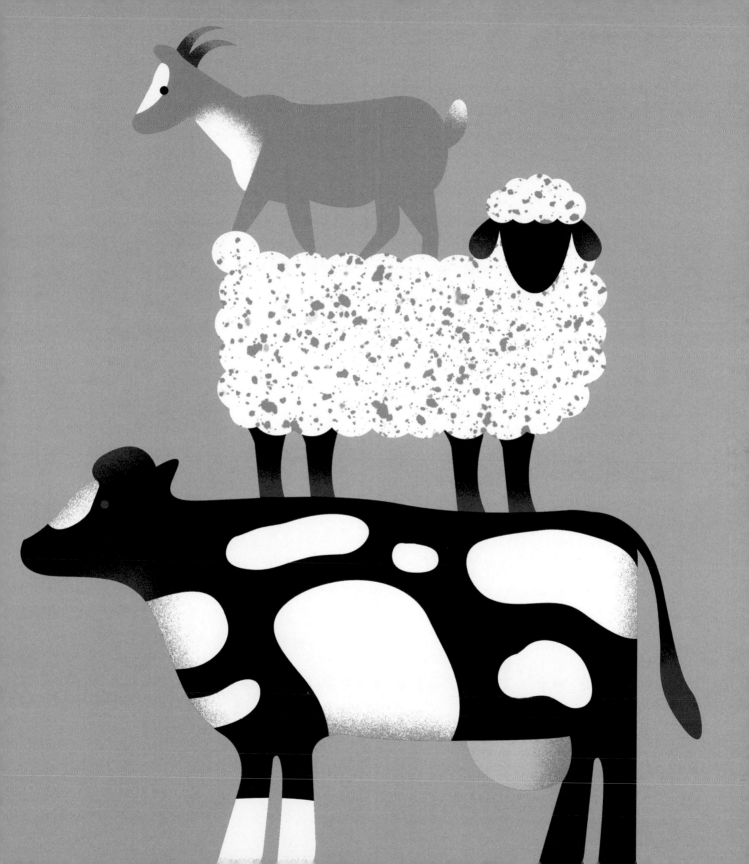

milk from a clean, trusted source, try it and see. (Turning it into yogurt or kefir will make it even more digestible.) I do recommend caution when buying raw soft cheeses.

I TOLERATE DAIRY JUST FINE!

That's great. As with any animal-sourced foods, the key is to up the quality and eat less of it. And always use whole-fat dairy, as low-fat versions rob you of nutrition and tend to be higher in sugars. To truly get the most benefits without the hazards, you'll need to read up on the brands you buy. Nutritionally speaking, the order of priority goes:

BEST: Raw dairy from grass-fed cows in safe/vetted facilities.

GOOD: Lightly pasteurized, non-homogenized whole milk from grass-fed cows, followed by lightly pasteurized, homogenized whole milk from grass-fed cows.

OKAY: Organic milk is legally required to come from cows that graze on grass or eat GMO-free grain without supplemental hormones or antibiotics. But recent investigations show some mega-dairies supplying your supermarket deny cows pasture, drastically lowering the "grass-fed" benefits of the milk. Check the Cornucopia Institute's Dairy Scorecard at cornucopia.org and learn about your sources.

WORST: Ultra-pasteurized, conventional nonfat milk.

And yes, doing dairy this way invariably costs more, so try the following:

REFRAME IT: See dairy as a condiment, the rich "accent" to a meal and an occasional, luxurious treat.

STRETCH IT: If you find rich and creamy grass-fed (or raw) milk, turn it into yogurt or kefir.

PRIORITIZE IT: Spend your pennies on grass-fed butter or ghee, which are concentrated sources of fat-soluble vitamins and protective fatty acids. "Cultured" butter is even better if you can find it!

JUST STOP IT: If higher-grade dairy is out of reach, consider using an organic dairy alternative, like nut or seed milks, instead.

Clinically, I've observed that dairy works well for many people, irritates others, and does violence to a few.

WHY TO SAY NO TO INDUSTRIAL DAIRY

Our modern sensitivities to dairy may be rooted less in the food itself and more in the industrialized way we now procure it. After all, for many peoples around the globe, this food is a dietary mainstay. Today we raise cows to produce three to four times more yield than they did one hundred years ago. Consider what goes into this:

The herbivore (naturally grass-eating) cows get fed grains. This puts GMOs and chemicals into their bodies and increases inflammatory omega-6 fatty acids.

The cows are regularly doctored with growth hormones (banned in Europe because they're considered disruptive to the endocrine system) and routinely administered antibiotics to fight the bacteria that spread in the close confines in which they live. They're also treated unethically and unnaturally.

Most milk, including organic, is pasteurized to reduce the high levels of pathogens that are pervasive in confined commercial dairies and to extend shelf life. These processes, especially Ultra-High Temperature (UHT) pasteurization, may change the components of milk, making casein less digestible, which prompts an inflammatory response. This could be why a large glass of milk may bother you more than, say, a swirl of kefir in your soup.

CHECK THE BOX

If you're buying boxed alternative milks, preferably look for ones that are organic, non-GMO, and unsweetened, with the shortest ingredient list possible. Avoid brands with carrageenan, a thickener made from seaweed that can trigger GI inflammation. And stay away from soy milk, a highly processed product that is known to disrupt endocrine function.

If dairy works for you, preferably choose full fat.

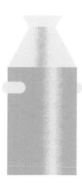

MAKE YOUR OWN NUT MILK

It's delicious. It's easy as pie. And it's liberating to replace boxed nut and seed milks—or "mylk" if you want to be trendy—with the fresh kind. You ditch unneeded sugars, preservatives, and thickening agents, and you get more nutrition from whole, barely processed ingredients. Use your straight-from-the-nut milk as a dairy substitute, or make it your base for smoothies or spiced-up hot chocolate. The easiest DIY milk to start with is almond, but once you've got that down, the options are endless—try cashews, hemp seeds, or shredded coconut milks next!

STEP 1: GATHER

You'll need 1 cup almonds or other nut, filtered water, a blender, either a piece of cheesecloth or a nut milk bag (easily sourced online), and a large bowl for draining the milk. Optional add-ins: 1 to 2 teaspoons cinnamon, a small splash of vanilla extract, or a scattering of Brazil nuts to ensure you get the all-important mineral selenium. Many recipes call for dates, which are tasty but unnecessary, especially since one large date can contain 16 grams of sugar! There's no reason that "milk" has to be sweet. (Note: If you don't have a top-of-the-line blender, dates will leave chunky bits in your drink).

STEP 2: SOAK

Place the nuts in your blender jar and cover with filtered water. Soak overnight; this helps make the nuts more digestible.

STEP 3: BLEND

The next morning, discard the soaking water, rinse the soaked nuts, and cover with 3 to 4 cups of filtered water (less water will make it creamier). Add any optional ingredients and blend well.

STEP 4: STRAIN

Pour the blended mixture through the cheesecloth or nut milk bag into your bowl. Squeeze to extract every last ounce of milk. Store in a clean, lidded glass jar in the fridge and use within 3 to 4 days. (Note: You can drink the milk without straining; it will just be grittier. Cashew milk does not need to be strained.)

After straining, you can save the ground nuts (aka "pulp") if you like. It's a coarser and less refined version of store-bought nut meal, useful for various baking and cooking recipes. Freeze in a baggie (no need to dry it first) until you're ready to use it.

OPTION: For a nut-free milk, blend ½ cup organic hulled hemp seeds with 4 cups water (no need to pre-soak the seeds). Flax seeds can also make an affordable seed milk (½ cup seeds to approximately 6 cups water). Soak the seeds for a few hours and rinse before blending and filtering as directed above. Flax milk is something of an acquired taste, so a little date and a splash of pure vanilla extract are warranted here.

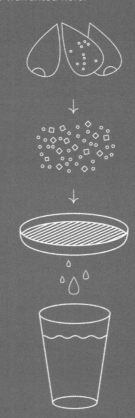

DON'T SWEAT **ABOUT SALT**

DON'T CHEAT YOURSELF OF SALT. IT'S AN ESSENTIAL MICRONUTRIENT THAT PLAYS A CRITICAL ROLE THROUGH- OUT YOUR BODY, HELPING TO REGULATE MUSCLE, HEART, NERVOUS SYSTEM, AND BRAIN FUNCTION; BLOOD FLOW; AND FLUID BALANCE. THOUGH SALT HAS GOTTEN A BAD RAP IN CONVENTIONAL MEDICINE, STRICT

CONTROL IS ONLY REQUIRED IN OCCASIONAL CASES. If you eat a clean, whole-foods diet and season your meals to taste, your body makes all the adjustments it needs to maintain equilibrium.

For optimal health, pay attention to the *kind* of salt you use. Unrefined salt (typically called sea salt) contains more than eighty valuable trace minerals that play essential roles in physiological functioning. Refined table salt has been bleached and baked into shimmering white crystals that lack these health aids. Pink Himalayan salt is considered the purest and best kind of unrefined salt—it comes from deep in the earth and is free of ocean contaminants—though most people tend to stick with less costly, coarse unrefined sea salt. Unfortunately, breaking research is revealing that plastics in the ocean are leaching into sea salt. Keep an eye on that story and consider diversifying your salts.

Signs that you've cut back too much on salt include low blood pressure, high stress, profuse sweating, and dehydration, as well as fatigue, cold extremities, decreased exercise performance, erectile dysfunction, sleep disturbances, and cognitive issues. Too little salt can even contribute to fat accumulation (it can dysregulate insulin).

The takeaway? Don't sweat it—eat whole foods and season them with unrefined salt to taste.

Dr. James DiNicolantonio is a leading cardiovascular research scientist and author of *The Salt Fix*. He shares the following thoughts:

HOW TO BE WELL EXPERT

1. **CONSCIOUSLY RESTRICTING SALT INTAKE IS CAUSING NEEDLESS SUFFERING.** I've found that many medications, disease states, and lifestyle choices cause us to need *more* salt, and if we would only listen to our internal salt hunger, we could start thriving again.

2. **SALT BECAME DEMONIZED BECAUSE OF ITS PREVALENCE IN PROCESSED FOODS.** But it's the mix of other ingredients—sugars, chemicals, heavy metals—in those foods that are the danger. Your body drives you to consume around 8 to 10 grams of salt each day, so if processed foods are engineered to be "low salt," you will likely end up eating *more* of them to get the salt your body craves. The unintended consequences of low-salt versions of processed foods (other than an increase in foodborne illnesses) is an increase in the risk of insulin resistance, diabetes, obesity, and overall cardiometabolic disease.

3. **REGULAR TABLE SALT IS HIGHLY PROCESSED AND LACKS MINERALS**, but you are better off consuming regular table salt than no salt at all. This is especially true of iodized salt, which delivers three essential minerals (iodine, sodium, and chloride).

>> **Unrefined sea salt contains more than eighty valuable trace minerals that play essential roles in physiological functioning.** <<

MAKE COOKING
IDIOT-PROOF

THE MORE YOU CAN GET IN THE GROOVE WITH COOKING AT HOME, THE MORE LIKELY YOU'LL EAT WELL. WHEN YOU COOK, YOU'RE SETTING YOURSELF UP TO WIN, BECAUSE STUDIES SHOW THAT THE MORE YOU COOK FROM SCRATCH, THE HIGHER YOUR STATE OF RESILIENCE AND FUNCTION. IF YOU DON'T COOK MUCH, IT CAN SEEM

INTIMIDATING, SO KEEP IT SIMPLE! ANYONE CAN COOK as long as they've shopped for food.

It's fairly easy to get a better breakfast; a Nourishing Smoothie (page 67) or some eggs over colorful vegetables couldn't be simpler. And lunch isn't difficult if you have good storage containers or jars and can commit to assembling components in advance (vegetables, canned wild salmon, organic turkey or chicken, hard-boiled eggs, and dressing). But dinner can overwhelm. Somehow, it feels more loaded—perhaps because of ideals from family members or foodie TV shows. Combine that with end-of-day inertia, and microwaved takeout or a cluster of snacks can become the default.

To turn that around, here are my health coaches' tactics for becoming captain of your cooking ship and getting homemade dinners on the table regularly.

LOWER THE BAR. If you barely cook, start with a goal of one or two homemade dinners a week. Begin with one basic meal you know you like—the simpler, the better—and make it a few times.

ISOLATE THE OBSTACLE. Do you forget to go shopping (page 73)? Are you too tired to prep in the evening? Or does the cleanup get you down? Know where you tend to trip up and do a time-audit: Where can you win back blocks of time to perform these tasks without stress? It might be a weekend afternoon or weeknight spent cooking in the kitchen with a glass of wine. Put it on your schedule.

INVEST IN A FEW VERY SIMPLE, TIME-SAVING TOOLS (see page 53). Arm yourself with a slow cooker or pressure cooker, and even with minimal experience, you can have large one-pot meals that can be portioned into individual servings (with extras for freezing). The ingredients can be prepped in advance, and the cooking happens while you're busy elsewhere. Find some of my favorite slow-cooker recipes at howtobewell.com

GO FOR BOWLS. Broths (see page 43) with added protein and vegetables become instant satisfying soup suppers, and roasted vegetables and cooked proteins give you the components to serve up the Perfect Plate (page 23) or bowl.

FREE YOURSELF FROM RECIPES. While most of us need recipes now and then, feeling dependent on recipes for every meal is a block to starting anything. Sticking to elemental plates and meals at first (grilled protein plus sides, pureed soups using vegetables you have on hand) will free you of this fear. Keep quality EVOO, salt, garlic, lemon, and a few spices in stock, and a recipe-free, vegetable-rich dinner can be made in twenty minutes.

ALWAYS COOK EXTRA AT DINNER. Leftovers make a great lunch the following day.

THINK RADICALLY. You give away your money and your power when you don't cook. Most restaurants and prepared foods use low-grade ingredients—it's about profit over health. Making your meals can save thousands of dollars a year, which you can put toward the truly health-building foods that you prep at home.

CONSIDER THE MEAL KIT. New delivery services offering boxes packed with ingredients for a home-prepped meal can be a stepping-stone when lack of time or expertise is stopping you short. There are plenty of them, from sunbasket.com to greenchef.com and more. It's still cooking, and once you get in a groove, the world is your oyster!

MAKE KITCHEN TIME FUN. Listening to a great podcast or music, or teaming up with friends or family to cook together, brings inspiration, education, and a few laughs into the mix.

GADGETS TO GET YOU CRUISING IN THE KITCHEN

SLOW COOKER: Great for soups, stews, slow-cooked meats and meat sauces, black beans, and daal

PRESSURE COOKER: A high-speed cooking instrument that can do everything the slow cooker does, and is especially quick for beans and legumes. It's even said to reduce the amount of "anti-nutrient" lectins in these foods, making them more digestible (page 37). The Instant Pot is a multifunction cooker that offers both pressure and slow options.

IMMERSION STICK BLENDER: Purees soups right in the pot, saving you time when you wash dishes

SPIRALIZER: Quickly makes vegetable noodles for steaming, sautéing, or using raw in salads

STEAMER POT: Essential for quick-cooked vegetables and reheating cooked proteins

KNIVES: A chef's knife and a paring knife are all you need

CHOPPING BOARDS: Use separate ones for meats and vegetables

CAST-IRON OR STAINLESS-STEEL PAN: For safely sautéing and cooking proteins and vegetables

VEGGIE BULLET: Treat yourself to this multifunction gadget if you want automated slicing, spiralizing, shredding, and blending

You can forge a more intimate relationship with food, demand integrity from food, and transform your health completely as a result — food is that powerful.

GIVE YOUR GUT
SOME LOVE

YOU PROBABLY KNOW YOU NEED SOME FERMENTED foods to feed and strengthen the biota in your belly, but are you actually eating them? Fermented foods are a health world manna—an inexpensive and reliable way to build up a healthy microbiome, an indispensable tool for strengthening your inner defenses, and often a kick-start to better digestion and elimination—but incorporating them into your diet can be awkward because the taste can take some getting used to. The flavor profile of most fermented foods (like raw sauerkraut and kimchi, its Korean counterpart, yogurt, kefir, kombucha, miso, and lacto-fermented pickles) is tart and sour, which are underdeveloped tastes to the Western palate and the opposite of the sweet profile that's come to dominate so many foods today. For most of us, cultured food is a taste we have to acquire and learn to love, bite by bite.

It's worth it. These humble power foods—made from basics like cabbage, carrots, radishes, tea, or plain and simple milk—really do build health from the inside out. And they add eclectic diversity to your diet. Fermented foods are unpredictable and colorful (just have a look at the Instagram feed @fermentationist for inspiration). When they're made the right way—left raw and unpasteurized so the active cultures can do their job—their tang provides a wild and unpredictable antidote to the homogeny of everyday eating.

It helps to know that these foods aren't intended to be eaten in giant amounts! They are condiments, served as a topping to your meal or a sidekick scoop to a protein, or in the case of beverages like kombucha, in small shots, not a pint glass.

I asked star chef **Seamus Mullen**, a close friend and author of the book *Real Food Heals*, for a few fermented food pairings: quick and tasty ways to integrate fermented foods into everyday

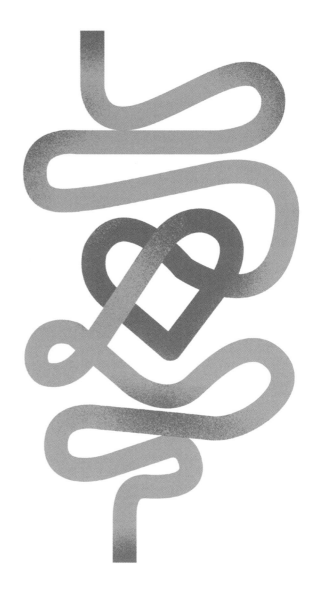

eating that also make meals a little more exciting. Using this list as a guide, commit to trying one new fermented food or drink this week.

SOUP: ADD A SWIRL OF KEFIR

Roast butternut squash in the oven, then scoop out the flesh and sauté it with olive oil, onion, garlic, ginger, and turmeric. Add chicken stock and simmer until everything is tender. Transfer to a blender and buzz with some kefir, salt and pepper to taste, and lime juice. Serve with chopped cilantro and mint.

SALAD: SPICE IT UP WITH KIMCHI

Puree kimchi into a silky marinade for grilled grass-fed beef or pastured chicken for dinner (marinate for at least 45 minutes or up to 8 hours), and then set some aside for a "live foods" vinaigrette dressing for a lunch salad. To make the dressing: Add ⅓ cup apple cider vinegar (also a fermented food) and ⅔ cup extra-virgin olive oil to 2 tablespoons pureed kimchi, then whisk with a pinch of sea salt. Assemble a salad of mustard greens, thinly sliced daikon or radish, avocado, sesame seeds, a sliced hard-boiled egg or two, and some excellent-quality anchovies or preserved tuna, and top with the dressing.

EGGS: HEAT THEM UP WITH FERMENTED CHILI PASTE

Scramble eggs in grass-fed ghee or butter. When serving, add a kick of heat with probiotic benefit: a dash of fermented chili sauce or fermented chili paste, which is easy and fun to make on your own if you don't want to buy it.

SALMON: DRESS IT UP WITH YOGURT

For an easy wild salmon dish, season a piece of salmon with sea salt, pepper, lemon zest, and a healthy dose of extra-virgin olive oil. Fold into a parchment-paper parcel with lots of fresh herbs (dill, tarragon, and basil). Bake in the oven at 350°F for 7 to 10 minutes. Meanwhile, prepare a tangy dressing by whisking together ⅔ cup full-fat yogurt, 1 grated garlic clove, 1 tablespoon lemon zest, 1 to

2 tablespoons extra-virgin olive oil, and cracked pepper, sea salt, and chopped fresh herbs to taste. Pour the dressing over the baked salmon and serve. (If your salmon piece serves only one or two people, use half of the dressing amount, or less.)

LAMB: BOOST THE NUTRITION WITH SAUERKRAUT

Make lamb burgers or meatballs, mixing spices, chopped nuts, and finely chopped greens directly into the ground meat. Serve with raw sauerkraut—the perfect complement to burgers (it will also work great with beef).

COCONUT: CREATE AN ADDICTING PROBIOTIC CREAM

Make your own coconut yogurt by adding yogurt or kefir cultures to coconut milk or coconut cream and fermenting it just like dairy. This fat-rich living food is delicious on its own with berries, or it can be thinned out to create vinaigrettes or add to soups and marinades.

6 MORE CULTURED FOODS TO TRY

- **PICKLES**
  Make sure they are unpasteurized, in brine, not vinegar

- **FERMENTED BEET JUICE**
  Also known as beet kvass

- **MISO PASTE**
  Made from soybeans, this is delicious in soups

- **WATER KEFIR OR COCONUT WATER KEFIR**
  A fizzy, low-sugar drink

- **SAUERKRAUT AND PICKLE JUICE**

- **LACTO-FERMENTED CONDIMENTS**
  Like salsa, homemade mayonnaise, and chutney

ALIVE AND KICKING

The "live" cultures of active probiotics found in fermented foods colonize your microbiome, helping to protect you from pathogens. They also release enzymes to ease and improve digestion (especially protein digestion) and make it easier for your body to extract and absorb more nutrients from your food. By promoting a well-balanced microbiome, they help with weight regulation by triggering "satiety" signals in your brain and helping with proper glucose and insulin regulation, and kimchi and sauerkraut in particular have anti-inflammatory wonder properties. They can even protect against depression and stress thanks to the gut-brain axis. Fermented foods and drinks might cause some gas—so start small and go slow. If you have digestive issues from an overgrowth of yeast (candida), you may have to clear that before adding these foods. (See "What to Do When . . ." on page 245.)

BUY OR DIY?

If you have more time than money, make your own fermented veggies using the small, countertop-size container from krautsource.com and buy starter cultures for kefir, yogurt, and more from culturesforhealth.com. If you have more money than time, shop for truly "live" fermented foods, not pasteurized ones, which kill the live cultures—they'll be in the refrigerated section of the grocery or health food store.

SOURDOUGH: A RETURN TO REAL BREAD?

Small-batch bakers are now making true sourdough again. In this traditional process, a mixture of wheat and rye flour is fermented for many hours (a minimum of four to six, and sometimes much longer) with a culture of wild yeast fungi and several strains of local lactobacilli, which breaks down the gluten proteins into digestible amino acids. The longer the ferment, the tangier the taste and, for those who are sensitive to gluten, the greater likelihood that you can enjoy small amounts of it. (Studies show that it doesn't spike blood sugar to the degree that regular wheat bread does.) The label for a *true* sourdough loaf will typically list some kind of sourdough starter or cultured flour, and no yeast (but not always; check your source and ask about their process).

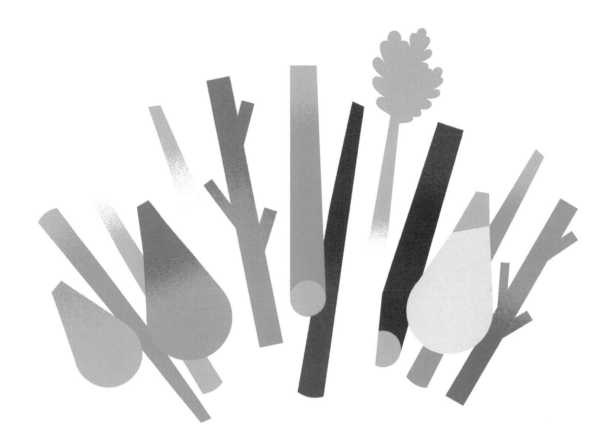

EAT THE STALKS **AND STEMS**

DON'T TOSS THAT STALK OF BROCCOLI OR THAT HEFTY CAULIFLOWER BASE! AND SAVE THOSE RIBBED RED STALKS OF CHARD AND SKINNY STEMS OF KALE OR COLLARD GREENS. THE TOUGH PARTS OF VEGGIES PLAY AN IMPORTANT ROLE IN HELPING THE HEALTH-PROTECTING MICROBES IN YOUR BELLY TO THRIVE. THEY CONTAIN

CELLULOSE FIBERS, HARD-TO-DIGEST CARBOHY-drates that give those good bacteria something to chew on. Fiber-rich foods like these (as well as woody asparagus stalks and stringy bits of celery) have prebiotic benefits: They work in tandem with probiotic foods to ensure a thriving microbiome. Consider them the fuel that feeds the probiotics, catalyzing them to do their work!

To use, slice stalks and stems into thin disks or skinny strips and throw them into your steamer or sauté pan alongside the more-celebrated parts of the vegetable. Munching on them raw—in moderation—confers even greater benefit (just don't go overboard, as this may give you gas). For the fullest prebiotic effect, add some of the following wonder foods to your daily regime: raw leeks, raw asparagus, raw dandelion leaves (added to salads), raw garlic, and raw or cooked onion.

GET YOUR VEG **TO 70%**

IF THERE IS ONE GAME-CHANGING ACTION YOU CAN START TODAY THAT WILL UTTERLY TRANSFORM YOUR STATE OF WELL-BEING, IT'S UPPING YOUR CONSUMPTION OF LIFE-SUPPORTING, PHYTOCHEMICAL-PACKED, MINERAL- AND VITAMIN-RICH, FIBER-LADEN VEGETABLES TO OPTIMAL LEVELS: AROUND TWO-THIRDS OF YOUR

FOOD INTAKE. 70 PERCENT SOUNDS IMPRESSIVE, I know. But it is quite achievable if you reverse your thinking and shift the green or crunchy portion of your meal from sidekick to starring role. You can do this by following the Perfect Plate (page 23) or simply repeating one of my favorite health mantras, picked up from Deborah Szekely, the founder of Rancho La Puerta, the very first health spa in the U.S.: *Make your main plate the side plate, and your side plate the main plate.* For optimal benefits, keep the starchiest sides, like potatoes, yams, and other tubers, to less than a quarter of the plate (and even less than that if you are going strictly low-carb; see page 84).

Does making this switch mean consuming buckets of salad every day? No. While salads are superb, vast quantities of raw vegetables are taxing to digest. And cooking vegetables often helps to release vital nutrients. I recommend borrowing the strategies of some of the savviest vegetable eaters I know. Implement one of these tactics every week, and within seven weeks your diet will be prolific with plants.

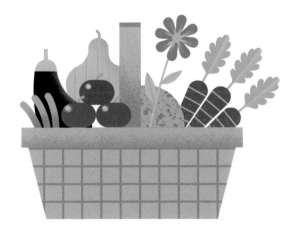

THE 10 HABITS OF SUCCESSFUL VEGETABLE EATERS

1. **THEY MAKE THEIR BED FIRST THING.** Make a layer of greens or mixed vegetables the foundation of every plate—include eggs or other proteins for breakfast! Steam or sauté with minced garlic, using EVOO and salt liberally.

2. **THEY SHOP, THEN PREP.** Bring home fresh produce and spend a few minutes prepping it so you can quickly grab fistfuls in the days ahead. Wash and dry salad and cooking greens well, then store in baggies with moisture-catching paper towels. Trim and chop cruciferous veggies like broccoli and cabbage so they're at the ready for steaming and sautéing. Slice up carrots, cucumbers, and peppers for quick crudité snacks.

3. **THEY ROAST FOR THE WEEK.** On your prep day or when you have a free twenty minutes, fill a roasting pan with chopped or whole cleaned sweet potatoes, beets, and squash. Fill another tray with a mix of Brussels sprouts and cauliflower or broccoli. Toss with a little olive oil and salt, then roast at 350°F until you can slide a knife in easily (for approximate times, download a chart at howtobewell.com). Use these over the next four to five days. Having these precious perishables precooked means you will waste far fewer of them.

4. **THEY MAKE SOUP.** Blend heaps of steamed vegetables with broth, salt, garlic, EVOO, and herbs, and presto, you'll drink more delicious vegetables than you could ever eat in one sitting. (In the heat of summer, you can also make chilled soups.)

5. **THEY REPLACE PASTA WITH SPIRALS AND STRANDS.** Make noodles from spiralized zucchini, winter squash, sweet potato, and more—a very light steam or quick sauté is all it takes. You can also roast a spaghetti squash and scoop out the strands. Or make kelp noodles—sea vegetables, available bagged in most health stores and some supermarkets—your "starchy" strings in warm and soupy broths. While you're at it, replace rice with the cauliflower kind—it also stands in as the basis for pizza crust (page 63).

6. **THEY ADD VEGETABLES TO EVERYTHING** (and go rogue with recipes). Look for any opportunity to stir spinach into a soup or sauce or scatter broccoli, mushrooms, and cauliflower into a curry or quinoa. Order that side of greens or a salad every time you eat out.

7. **THEY MASTER THE MEAL HACK.** Make your too-busy-to-cook dinner staple a bowl of broth with abundant fresh or frozen vegetables and whisked-in egg or other proteins. A dash of liquid aminos or tamari for flavor, and it's go time.

8. **THEY STOCK THE FREEZER.** Fill it with several kinds of frozen organic vegetables so you never lack the materials for a veggie-filled meal.

9. **THEY EAT IN TECHNICOLOR.** Use produce to add more colors to your bowl: purple cabbage, orange carrots, red peppers. When you add more colors, you get more protective phytochemicals.

10. **THEY FOLLOW GOOD HASHTAGS.** The new eater-friendly trends break on social media. Sweet potato toast instead of grains? That's just the start. Follow a few feeds like @willfrolicforfood and @ohsheglows, or some of the colorful vegan-oriented feeds. Some of these use considerable grains and sugars, but if you pick your inspiration wisely, you can tap into infinite crafty ways to vegify your diet.

Eat the right foods and they will send instructions to your genes for good health. Eating the wrong foods, however, sends messages for disease.

◄◄

BECOME A
REAL-FOOD SNACKER

MY PATIENTS ARE OFTEN SURPRISED TO FIND OUT THAT SNACKS ARE NOT TABOO. HEALTHY EATING DOES NOT HAVE TO MEAN GOING HUNGRY. EATING BETWEEN MEALS IS OKAY IF YOU ARE LEGITIMATELY HUNGRY (AND NOT BORED/ANTSY/DRIVEN TO DISTRACTION, BECAUSE SNACKING IS A RED FLAG OF MINDLESS AND EMOTION-

CHARGED EATING). INTERESTINGLY, WHEN YOUR DIET is upgraded—liberated from processed foods and freed of excess carbs—your dependence on snacks tends to lessen. You're getting more nutrition from your food, so you feel more sated.

When you do need some help bridging the gap between meals, please don't snack on supersized, flavor-engineered bags of chips or pretzel sticks (or worse, vending machine candy). Seize the chance to fuel yourself on actual nutrition, with real fats and quality proteins snuck into the mix. Whether you make or buy your snack food (hint: one of those is cheaper), lean on real foods as the foundation—no junk seed oils and added sugars! Lace your snacks with surprising flavor and sprinkle them with functional or medicinal ingredients if you like. Here are five healthy contenders on the modern snack landscape, all of which give you good nutritional bang for each bite.

THE NEW NUTRITION BAR: Energy balls have retired the syrupy, fructose-laden, processed-GMO-soy bar of yore. Easy to DIY, they combine nut meals and butters with protein powders, a touch of raw honey or dates, and add-ins galore, from shredded coconut, cacao, goji berries, and chia seeds to spirulina and spices. (They can even carry adaptogens like maca powder or medicinal mushrooms, page 45, so with practice you can make a ball to target your unique needs!) The energy ball is a close relative to the fat bomb, the bites beloved by low-carb and ketogenic eaters. *Tip: Use the almond meal from your homemade almond milk!*

THE WILD ONES: Jerky and its close cousin, the primal meat bar, have changed the game of snacking (and made sugar-filled granola bars obsolescent). Look for brands made from 100 percent grass-fed meat, free of sugars and additives like MSG and fake flavors. Meat bars have more fat content than jerky, making them moist, chewy, and curiously satisfying. (Some brands, like Pure Traditions, even contain organ meats, helping to fill modern nutritional gaps.) If you're up for adventure, seek out my "jerky" of choice, the South African version, biltong (which I used to make while working as a doctor in the South African bush); the grass-fed kind is available at braaitime. com or biltongusa.com. *Tip: Shred some jerky into trail mix you make yourself (from raw and unsalted nuts and seeds). Add a few goji berries and you're ready to run.*

THE DAILY FIX: Make raw vegetables and low-sugar fruits—cut up and ready to go—the cornerstone of your snack supplies. Pair them with something that adds some good fat: thin kohlrabi slices with EVOO-rich hummus; cucumber with goat cheese and avocado or even smoked fish; or green apple or celery with sugar-free, oil-free nut butter. Better yet, make it fermented: A pickle with hummus or a hard-boiled egg with sauerkraut will refresh your palate as it fuels your energy.

SUPPORTING PLAYERS

THE RENEGADE: One hundred percent gluten-free and seed-oil-free crackers have won legions of fans, plus they're one of the most benevolent gluten-free packaged foods, as they use no industrial oils or fillers (the ones made by Mary's Gone Crackers are a good example). Now, for those avoiding common inflammatory foods like corn, grain-free tortilla chips from companies like The Real Coconut and

Siete Foods are hitting the scene with tortillas and chips made of coconut flour or cassava flour and heat-tolerant coconut or avocado oil—not exactly health food, but a giant step forward from Doritos.

THE DIVA: Raw, sprouted, stone-ground nut butters from small-batch makers like Jem Organics might use pecans, pistachios, pumpkin seeds, and more, fused with delicious spices and superfood ingredients. Think of them as your indulgence—they are spendy, but delicious.

Your body responds to processed foods as if they are "foreign bodies," prompting an inflammatory response as it tries to protect itself.

◄◄

CHOCOLATE ENERGY BALLS

- 1 cup leftover almond "pulp" (from making almond milk) or 1 cup almond flour
- 1 cup shredded unsweetened coconut flakes
- ½ cup almond butter or coconut butter
- 3 tablespoons coconut oil (room temperature or softened over low heat)
- 3 heaping tablespoons cacao powder
- 3 tablespoons cacao nibs
- 3 tablespoons hemp seeds
- 2 tablespoons ground almond meal (store-bought)
- 1 tablespoon pure vanilla extract, or more to taste
- Few pinches cinnamon, to taste
- Up to 2 tablespoons maple syrup to sweeten, optional

Add all the ingredients to your food processor and process until it's the consistency of fudge; taste and add more cinnamon and vanilla if needed, to suit your preference. If you use the maple syrup, add just a little to start—you may not need as much as you think—and then add more dry ingredients if necessary to achieve a fudge-like consistency. Roll the mixture into small balls and store in a sealed container in the fridge for up to 2 weeks, or in the freezer for up to 2 months.

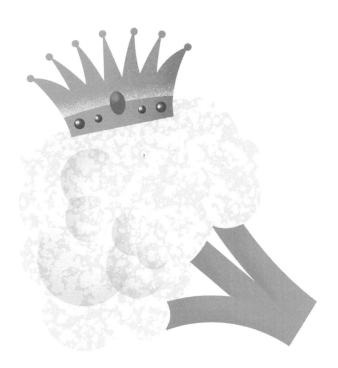

LET THEM EAT
CAULIFLOWER!

THE HUMBLE CAULIFLOWER MIGHT NOT MAKE HEADLINE NEWS, BUT IN THE WORLD OF WELLNESS IT'S A LOW-CARB DARLING: A NUTRITIOUS AND ANTIOXIDANT-RICH VEGETABLE THAT FULFILLS THE URGE FOR STARCHY SATISFACTION FROM POTATOES, PASTA, AND RICE, WHILE SPARING YOUR BLOOD SUGAR THE IMPACT

OF THAT STARCH. IT IS ALSO INCREDIBLY VERSATILE, pleasingly affordable, and so easy to use, and in such a variety of ways, that I consider it a gateway vegetable, one of those staple foods that starts to help you shift from packaged noodles or high-carb potatoes to the place where vegetables form the healthful base of each meal.

Whatever your past associations with this hearty vegetable may be, there are no more reasons to call it bland. The genius of cauliflower is that it holds up well to all kinds of transformations: mash it with butter or blitz it into puree; roast its tasty crowns (at 425°F for 20 minutes, stirring occasionally), or snack on it raw. You can even scatter it into stir-fries or (if you're ambitious) shape the pulverized rice—see How to Make Cauliflower Rice (opposite)—into

trendy cauliflower-crust pizza. Or just steam and serve: The textured crowns catch drizzles of oil and sauces like Bolognese and sprinkles of health-enhancing spices brilliantly.

Commit to using one cauliflower per week and it will not only fill you with its phytochemical content, it will transform the way you see your plate. The next thing you know, you'll be making Swiss chard for breakfast without a second thought.

Buy smart: Cauliflower fills your plate with good nutrition at a very reasonable price. It's not imperative to buy organic—the Environmental Working Group has cauliflower on its "Clean 15" list—but if you can find organic, all the better.

HOW TO MAKE CAULIFLOWER RICE

THIS IS ABOUT AS EASY AS COOKING COMES. THE "RICE" GOES well with all kinds of dishes, from curries to roasted veggies to your favorite protein and more. You can use fresh cauliflower, but precut, frozen cauliflower will work fine. And if you find green, orange, or purple cauliflower, have fun with them. (The colors bring their own unique health-protecting phytonutrients.)

STEP 1 Gather your materials.

- 1 medium head cauliflower (fresh or frozen)
- 2 tablespoons coconut oil or grass-fed butter
- 1 small onion, peeled and diced
- Sea salt and freshly ground pepper to taste

STEP 2 Rinse and dry the cauliflower, then cut the florets into big pieces and slice the thick stalk into thin disks.

STEP 3 Working in batches, put a few pieces of the cauliflower into a food processor and pulse until it is crumbly and resembles rice. Continue with the remaining pieces. You can also do this by grating with a cheese grater.

STEP 4 Heat the coconut oil or butter in a large pan, add the onion, and sauté until the onion is lightly browned. Add the "riced" cauliflower and sauté until it is cooked through but not mushy (think al dente), about 8 minutes. Season to taste with salt and pepper.

SPICE IT UP Add a special kick of colorful and flavorful spices. Halfway through sautéing the onion, add the following and stir frequently: 1 clove minced garlic, ½ teaspoon cumin, ½ teaspoon turmeric, and ½ teaspoon ground ginger.

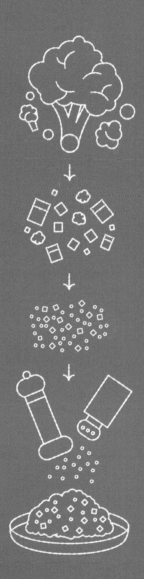

BECOME A CACAO
CONNOISSEUR

CHOCOLATE IS THE TREAT THAT I HAVE FEW QUALMS PRESCRIBING. FOR MILLENNIA, MESOAMERICAN CUL-TURES KNEW IT AS HERBAL MEDICINE AND SACRED FOOD—A COMPONENT OF CEREMONY AND A "FOOD OF THE GODS." TODAY WE KNOW IT AS A KIND OF BITTERSWEET MULTIVITAMIN CAPABLE OF REDUCING OXIDATIVE STRESS

(A ROOT CAUSE OF ILLNESS AND AGING), COUNTERing inflammation and lowering blood pressure, and boosting mental focus and cognitive longevity. We're coming full circle back to the sacred part, too. You don't need to be a scientist to know that really good chocolate, mindfully eaten, can induce waves of optimism and calm.

That happy feeling doesn't come because it is sweet. It's born of the vital ingredient: the cacao. Get into the habit of taking modest (one to two small squares) daily doses of super-quality chocolate—the kind that's undergone as little processing as possible—and, assuming you aren't sensitive to this stimulant, you can truly get all of the pleasure with none of the guilt. Here's the lowdown on how chocolate is made so you can suss out which bars are best.

THE REAL CHOCOLATE STORY:
FROM BEAN TO BAR

1. **THE BEANS ARE GROWN IN REGIONS CLOSE TO THE EQUATOR.** The seeds of the *Theobroma cacao* tree (from the Greek for "food of the gods"), cacao beans are nestled inside football-shaped pods on the tree. Cacao is abundant in chemicals produced by the body but rarely found in foods, like anandamide (a bliss-inducing hormone you normally produce after exercise). Treat this queen of plant foods with some respect by buying chocolate from ethical makers. A "Fair Trade" stamp is a good indicator, though "Direct Trade" benefits the cacao farmer even more.

2. **BEANS ARE HARVESTED, FERMENTED, DRIED, AND ROASTED.** The beans become cocoa nibs—bitter and intense, bursting with beneficial flavonoids and essential minerals like magnesium. Try using this crunchy power food in smoothie bowls or chia puddings, or eat it on its own as an energizing snack. You can drink ground roasted beans (from brands like Crio Bru) like coffee—just steep and sip. The theobromine delivers a sustained lift without the caffeine jitters. (Note: "Raw" chocolate, which is processed at lower temperatures, claims to have the highest antioxidant levels of all.)

3. **NIBS ARE GROUND, MIXED INTO A PASTE, AND SEPARATED FROM COCOA BUTTER TO DELIVER COCOA SOLIDS.** Sugar is added at this stage to balance the bitter taste, but there's no need for the supersweet ratio of mass-market chocolate. Go low, with a bar touting at least 75 percent cacao content. (The

>>

Fall in love with cacao and boost your happy chemical, serotonin, naturally.

<<

higher the number, the "darker" and more intense the chocolate, and the lower the sugar.) And look for dairy-free: Some studies say that the milk (or milk powder) present in chocolate, even in many dark chocolate brands, will bind with the antioxidants and prevent full absorption.

4. **THE CHOCOLATE-SUGAR MIX UNDERGOES CONCHING AND TEMPERING AND BECOMES . . . A CHOCOLATE BAR!** Check how many ingredients are listed—the fewer the better. The best dark chocolate always has chocolate liquor or cocoa listed as the first ingredient (and may also list cocoa powder, cocoa nibs, and cocoa butter), with sugar at the end. Take a taste and notice the flavor: With few supporting players, you'll enjoy discovering all kinds of cacao nuances, just like with wine.

5. **NEW-WAVE ADD-INS BOOST THE BAR FURTHER.** Artisanal chocolatiers are going wild with superfood and medicinal add-ins, using anything from spices and medicinal mushrooms to (yes) kale chips to give the bar extra-good properties and keep all your senses engaged. Get adventurous (but choose organic—dubious suppliers can sneak in all kinds of unwanted additives under the "flavors" tag).

6. **A JAZZY LOGO, AND A HIGHER-THAN-AVERAGE PRICE TAG, ADD THE FINAL TOUCH.** You have in your hands a functional-food luxury. Treat your (sweetish) treat with reverence. Savor it, one small brick at a time. Chocolate is a renowned food for mindful eating practices—commit to using it that way by slowing down and sinking into the experience, becoming fully present with how it changes the way you feel and think.

A FEW OF MY FAVORITE BRANDS:

- Madécasse (madecasse.com)
- Raaka (raakachocolate.com)
- Wei (weiofchocolate.com)
- Kakawa (for exceptional drinking elixirs; kakawachocolates.com)

Eating sugar triggers hormones that signal fat cells to store fat, whereas fat does not trigger the same hormones.

PRACTICE EATING MINDFULLY

1 Slow down

2 Sit down

3 Breathe

4 Look at your food

5 Take it all in—colors, shapes, textures

6 Smell it

7 Bless it

8 Breathe

9 Look at your food

10 Take a bite

11 Chew slowly and consciously

12 Taste your food

13 Relish your food

14 Sip small sips of your drink, not gulps

15 Keep tasting your food

16 Check in midway: Am I still hungry?

17 Stop when you're 80 percent sated

18 Notice how you feel now

PRACTICE SNACKING MINDFULLY

1 Ask the question: Am I hungry?

2 Or is it something else?

3 Boredom?

4 Discomfort?

5 Longing?

6 Have a glass of water

7 Wait two minutes

8 Ask yourself again: Am I hungry?

9 If yes, eat and enjoy

MASTER THE
NOURISHING SMOOTHIE

THE NOURISHING SMOOTHIE IS LIKE A LIQUID FORM OF THE PERFECT PLATE (PAGE 23): IT IS BOOSTED WITH QUALITY FATS FOR SUSTAINED ENERGY AND HEALTHY METABOLISM, STRENGTHENED BY GOOD PROTEINS (WHETHER PLANT- OR ANIMAL-BASED), AND, AS A FINAL TOUCH, CUSTOMIZED WITH MEDICINAL BOOSTERS, BE

THEY SIMPLE SPICES, ADAPTOGENS, OR SUPERFOOD powders. It can fuel you for hours and deserves the title of liquid meal. (It's also easy on the digestion, good for when you're feeling sluggish and need to give your system a break.) This is not your old-school "sugar bomb" smoothie, filled with sweet fruits and juices.

Use this basic formula to make a spectrum of different smoothies. Pick one ingredient from each tier or two from tiers 2, 3, and 4. If you want specific recipes, see page 68 for a few ideas, and you can find many more on howtobewell.com. But since smoothies are really all about freestyling—no exact measurements required—do some trial-and-error experiments and find your own favorites (they may not always taste of perfection, but the ingredients will be good for you).

You'll notice that most fruity ingredients are left out of these blends; this is to keep sugars low. You won't see fruit juices and tropical fruits like pineapple and mango. Even bananas, which are high in carbohydrates, are missing; we substitute new-wave smoothie concepts like cauliflower or creamy avocado. If you're going to use fruit, berries, which are low in sugars, are the way to go, but try going fruit-free, too.

Because this smoothie is a meal in a cup, don't gulp it down as you rush from point A to point B. Try to "chew" it rather than guzzle it (this helps digestion), and consume it as mindfully as you would any other lovingly prepared food. And consuming it at room temperature is easier on the digestion than drinking it icy cold.

TIER 1: LIQUID BASE ($\frac{1}{2}$ TO 2 CUPS)

- Nondairy milk (almond, coconut, hemp—avoid soy and rice)
- Organic unsweetened yogurt or kefir thinned with water
- ¼ cup raw, unflavored coconut water + ¾ cup water (to reduce the sugar)
- Optional add-ins:
    - Berries (fresh or frozen, up to ⅓ cup)
    - Spinach and other leafy greens (up to 1 cup)
    - Cauliflower (fresh or frozen; up to ½ cup)
    - Juice from 1 lime (best for green smoothies)

TIER 2: FAT ($\frac{1}{4}$ CUP TO $\frac{1}{2}$ CUP)

- ¼ to ½ avocado, fresh or frozen
- Full-fat coconut milk
- Unsweetened coconut yogurt
- ¼ cup nut butter (except peanut butter or peanut butter powder—peanuts commonly have mold toxicity)
- ¼ cup seed butter, such as tahini
- 1 to 2 tablespoons coconut butter, coconut oil, or MCT oil (a specialty concentrated oil derived from coconut)
- 1 to 2 tablespoons flax or chia seeds (Note: chia seeds tend to have higher lectin content)

TIER 3: PROTEIN (1 SERVING, PER DIRECTIONS ON THE PACKAGE)

- Collagen powder
- Protein powder like grass-fed whey, organic pea, or organic hemp
- 2 to 3 tablespoons organic hemp seeds

TIER 4: SPICE OR SUPERFOOD

- 1 tablespoon maca powder: for strength, hormone balance, and energy
- 1 tablespoon cacao powder or nibs: for focus, alertness, and extra antioxidants
- 1 teaspoon spirulina: for detoxification, energy boost, and plant protein
- 1 teaspoon chlorella: for immune and detoxification support
- 2 tablespoons goji berries: for antioxidants
- Half a pack of unsweetened frozen açai or 1 teaspoon açai powder: for antioxidants and healthy fats
- 1 teaspoon elderberry powder or half a dropper elderberry tincture: for immune support
- 1 scoop greens powder: for vitamins, minerals, anti-inflammatory effects, and immunity support
- ¼ teaspoon ground cinnamon: for balanced blood sugar and immunity support
- ⅛ teaspoon ground turmeric: for anti-inflammatory effects
- Sprinkle of bee pollen: for energy, allergy remedy, and plant protein
- Pinch of sea salt: for electrolytes
- Serving of powdered probiotics: for microbiome support
- 2 to 4 drops stevia or vanilla stevia: if needed for sweetness (alcohol-free; look for a brand that contains no added fillers)

When buying ingredients, look for organic, raw, and sustainably sourced.

PUTTING IT ALL TOGETHER

Here are some of my favorite smoothie recipes:

CHOCOLATE ENERGY

This is my morning go-to—and how I start every day.
- 1 serving vanilla protein powder (preferably whey from grass-fed cows)
- ¾ cup unsweetened coconut milk

- ¼ cup brewed organic coffee or 1 teaspoon organic instant coffee powder (optional)
- 1 to 2 tablespoons raw cacao
- ¼ avocado
- 1 tablespoon almond butter
- 1 tablespoon coconut oil
- 1 tablespoon flax, hemp, or chia seeds
- ¼ teaspoon ground cinnamon
- 6 to 8 ice cubes or approximately ½ cup room-temperature water

MORNING FUEL

- 1 cup almond milk
- ½ cup frozen blueberries
- 1 tablespoon coconut oil
- 1 teaspoon bee pollen
- 1 tablespoon almond butter
- 1 serving vanilla protein powder or 1 serving collagen powder + 2 to 4 drops vanilla stevia

GREEN DETOX

- 1 cup unsweetened coconut milk
- 1 teaspoon spirulina or 1 teaspoon chlorella (or ½ teaspoon of each)
- Juice from ½ lime
- 1 tablespoon coconut oil
- 1 tablespoon chia seeds
- 1 serving vanilla protein powder or collagen powder + 2 to 4 drops stevia (optional)
- Optional protein
- Ice and water

GOLDEN MILK SMOOTHIE

- 1 cup unsweetened coconut milk
- 1 teaspoon ground turmeric
- ¼ teaspoon ground ginger or ¼-inch piece peeled fresh ginger
- ½ orange, peeled, seeded, and chopped
- 1 tablespoon coconut oil
- 1 serving vanilla protein powder
- A few ice cubes

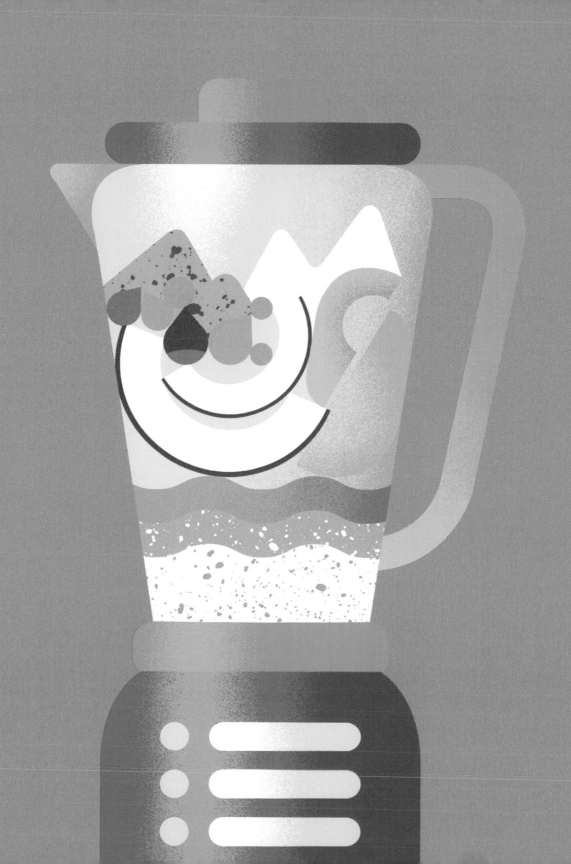

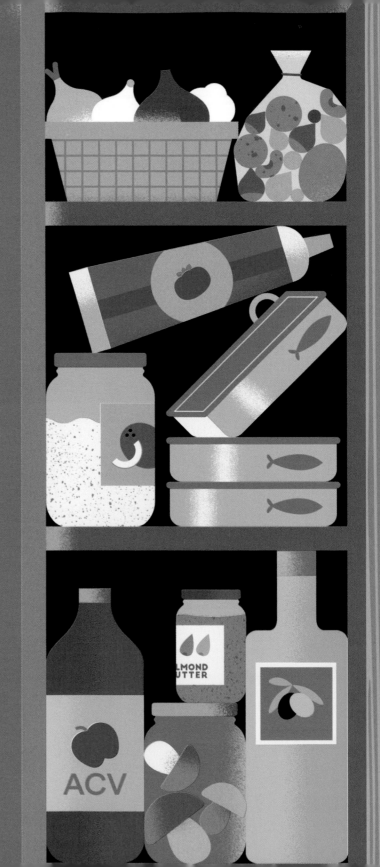

ORGANIZE YOUR
FRIDGE AND PANTRY

BUILDING A FUNCTIONAL SYSTEM FOR YOUR PROVISIONS ISN'T EXACTLY SEXY (UNLESS SPATIAL ORGANIZA- TION FLOATS YOUR BOAT), BUT IT IS THE ROBUST AND RELIABLE BACKBONE OF HEALTHY EATING. WHEN YOUR REFRIGERATOR AND PANTRY ARE STOCKED WITH REAL FOODS THAT CAN BE COOKED SIMPLY AND FAST, YOU

WON'T FLAIL IN THE FACE OF HUNGER AND FALL INTO the take-out (or chips for dinner) trap. Use these templates—based on the fridges and pantries of myself and my health coaches—as motivation to help you implement your own system for staying supplied. You might prefer to do big restock shopping sessions or incrementally add to your stash, buying as the need (or recipe) demands—either way works.

The goal here is not to build a Pinterest-worthy pantry. It's to get beyond that sad state when your kitchen is a barren wasteland, or a jumble of well-intentioned purchases that never quite get used, both of which are pitfalls to healthy eating. The motto is, "If you buy it, and if you can see it, you will eat it."

FRIDGE

BOTTOM VEGETABLE DRAWERS

LEFT SIDE: Salad and cooking greens, cruciferous vegetables (such as broccoli, cauliflower, radish, and kale), parsley
RIGHT SIDE: Green apples, various vegetables that were priced right this week

LOWER SHELF
- Roasted chicken, pastured eggs, meatballs (ready to eat), organic tempeh (for vegetarians)

MIDDLE SHELF
- Cooked quinoa, rice, root vegetables
- Chopped fruit
- Broths
- Nut milks

CHEESE DRAWER
- Goat cheese, grass-fed butter
- Tasty vegan cheese for the dairy-free (easy to DIY, or brands like Kite Hill)
- Grain-free wraps

TOP SHELF
- Yogurt (milk or coconut)
- Sauerkraut and pickles
- Hummus
- Energy balls
- Chia pudding

FRIDGE DOOR SHELVES
- Sugar-free ketchup, mustard, flax oil, olives
- Probiotic salad dressing—homemade!
- Ginger and turmeric—stored in paper bags
- Organic miso paste

FREEZER

- Vegetables—spinach, broccoli, cauliflower
- Berries
- Avocado chunks (for smoothies)
- Premade stews and soups, precooked beans
- Ground beef or lamb, or other cuts
- Chicken
- Wild salmon
- Coconut ice cream—a low-sugar treat—or homemade ice pops (freeze your smoothie of choice in ice pop molds)

PANTRY

- Coconut oil, ghee, lard
- Vinegars, Bragg Liquid Aminos, curry paste
- Raw honey (use in moderation)
- Dried or canned beans and legumes
- Pseudo-grains (if you eat them): quinoa, buckwheat, amaranth
- Nuts and seeds, nut butters, tahini
- Boxed alternative milk and canned coconut milk
- Canned sardines, mackerel, wild salmon
- Canned tomatoes and tomato paste
- Spice rack
- Salts and seaweed
- Garlic and onions, root vegetables, beets
- Organic teas and coffees
- Green powders, cacao, and protein powders

When you eat, you're not just feeding yourself; you're also providing meals to the trillions of microbes that live in your gut.

STOCK YOUR SHELVES
(WITHOUT STRESSING OUT)

THE DIFFERENCE BETWEEN PEOPLE WHO EAT WELL EVERY DAY AND THOSE WHO DON'T? ONE GROUP MAKES SHOPPING A NONNEGOTIABLE PART OF THEIR ROUTINE. IT'S A TRIED-AND-TRUE LAW: IF GOOD FOOD'S NOT STOCKED IN THE KITCHEN, YOU'LL PROBABLY EAT BADLY. FOLLOW THESE TOP TEN TIPS FOR MAKING IT HAPPEN—WEEK IN AND WEEK OUT.

SHOP SIMPLY. Don't obsess about mastering new recipes. Buy staple ingredients on repeat.

SKIP THE LINES, SKIP THE STRESS, AND SKIP THE TEMPTATIONS. Try online grocery delivery services like insta cart.com, shipt.com, or AmazonFresh (or local organic-shopping services like the Bay Area's goodeggs.com). Membership-based health-food retailer thrivemarket.com can help you stock your pantry affordably (its app can keep you stocked in basics, and its products are 100 percent GMO-free). Use specialty providers like grassland-beef.com, and butcherbox.com for high-quality grass-fed meat, and vitalchoice.com and sea2table.com for fish. One of the Be Well team's favorite aids for locating local sources of grass-fed meat, eggs, and dairy is eatwild.com.

BUY FRESH PRODUCE AT THE FARMERS' MARKET. The time saved by strategic online ordering can be diverted to this essential strategy to ensure your kitchen is loaded with fruits, vegetables, and herbs.

MAKE LISTS. Either old-school (with a whiteboard on the fridge or a pad and pen), or digital, using shopping apps like AnyList that let multiple people share lists. Some apps, like BigOven and Buy Me a Pie!, integrate recipes and meal planning into the lists.

TAKE 20 MINUTES TO PLOT OUT THE MAIN MEALS FOR EACH WEEK. This cuts down on trips to the store and reduces anxiety as the days fly by. Hanging a colorful chart on the fridge can get kids engaged in the act of preparing food.

JOIN TOGETHER. Becoming a member of a food co-op provides good prices on healthy and organic foods as well as a sense of community. Joining a CSA (community-supported agriculture) program ensures fresh local produce every week. While you're at it, why not share a cow from a local ranch?

BUY IN BULK. Source nuts, seeds, grains, beans, lentils—i.e., food without labels—in the bulk section at health-food stores and at some bigger supermarkets with organic sections. As long as they're freshly restocked, and ideally organic, these affordable buys can help save money over prepackaged versions.

COMPARE PRICES. Use price-tracking apps like Grocery iQ and discount stores and wholesale clubs like Costco.

DON'T BUY BOTTLED DRINKS OF ANY KIND (ESPECIALLY WATER). Why blow the budget on beverages when you can make your own teas and tonics? (See page 110.)

BRING YOUR OWN SHOPPING BAGS. Because it's the right thing to do.

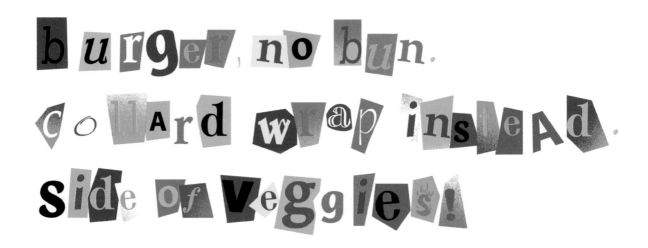

burger, no bun.
collard wrap instead.
side of veggies!

HACK THE **MENU**

IF YOU EAT OUT FREQUENTLY, YOU HAVE TO TREAT RESTAURANTS LIKE YOUR KITCHEN. GET SAVVY ABOUT HACKING THE MENU TO MAKE A MEAL THAT SKEWS CLOSER TO THE PERFECT PLATE (PAGE 23)—WITH VEGETABLES CROWDING OUT STARCHES, AND MODERATE PORTIONS OF PROTEIN—AND CONSIDER WHAT'S BEING USED TO

PREPARE YOUR MEAL. FRIED FOOD WILL ALMOST always deliver a dose of heated seed oils (see page 76), and if you're avoiding gluten, it will often be hidden in sauces. Some restaurants—like made-to-order salad chains or the growing number of grass-fed-burger joints—make all of this easier. Then there are farm-to-table places using fresh local ingredients—those are a no-brainer. But if picking the place isn't in your control, don't stress (because stress shuts down your digestion). Sharing a meal is also about communing and relating, so enjoy the company

and use these tested menu hacks to keep your healthier eating on track.

MEXICAN

Go for the fajitas (shrimp, chicken, beef, or just vegetables) with salsa or pico de gallo and (definitely!) guacamole, but leave items made with wheat and GMO-laden corn tortillas alone. *Hacking Tip:* Order a double salad with grilled chicken or shrimp, topped with avocado or guacamole. Add a small portion of beans if you are not strictly counting carbs and/or are vegetarian.

JAPANESE

Steer clear of fried tempura and dishes with heavy sauces; instead, opt for simple sushi rolls or sashimi (the guide on seafoodwatch.org can help you order sustainably). Choose tamari, which is a gluten-free soy sauce, if they offer it. *Hacking Tip:* Naruto rolls are wrapped in cucumber instead of rice—helpful if you're avoiding grains—and if you're avoiding lectins, go for white rice if given a choice.

STEAKHOUSE

Scour the side dishes for vegetables and double up on those—giving them the bulk of the plate—and split an oversize steak or burger (skipping the bun) with someone else. Pass on anything cheesy, fried, or breaded (sorry, onion rings). *Hacking Tip:* Choose any type of fish or animal protein you like and pair it with vegetables and/or salad.

ITALIAN

Be wary of the heavy bowl of pasta, especially if you're cutting gluten or lowering carbs. Avoid the bread basket, too, but if you *do* have a slice, eat it mindfully, savoring each bite! Grilled or roasted fish or meat, a salad, and a side of sautéed vegetables like spinach or broccoli rabe are surefire winners. *Hacking Tip:* An appetizer of mussels marinara paired with a salad and veggies makes a complete meal.

BURGERS AND PIZZA

Wrap the burger in lettuce, sub salad for fries, and (no surprise) nix the soda. For pizza, load on vegetable toppings, stick to one slice, and get a large salad on the side. *Hacking Tip:* Gluten-free pizza, if you're sensitive,

is increasingly common, and so is vegan cheese for the dairy-sensitive. I don't consider it healthy—but if the occasion calls for it, eat and enjoy.

VIETNAMESE

For a lighter alternative to Chinese food with its sugary, starchy sauces, load up broth-based pho with vegetables and your meat of choice. Rice noodles are used instead of wheat (so no gluten for the averse), and fresh cilantro and mint aid digestion. *Hacking Tip:* Green papaya salad and fresh rice-paper-wrapped vegetable rolls round out your meal.

CLASSIC DELI

If this is your lunch option, make sure to peruse the cold sides like broccoli rabe and vegetable salads. Instead of sandwiches, look for soups. If they roast their own meats (like turkey), combine that with salads to make a plate. *Hacking Tip:* Ask for sandwich proteins served on a bed of arugula or mixed greens instead of bread.

Check out cleanplates.com for news on new casual restaurants and what they're serving.

When it comes to calories, focus more on the quality than the quantity.

GET YOUR OIL CHANGED

NOTHING IN YOUR KITCHEN NEEDS WISER CURATION THAN YOUR COLLECTION OF COOKING AND POURING OILS. NOT ALL OILS ARE CREATED EQUAL—AND NOT ALL COOK EQUALLY, EITHER. SOME FATS ARE ROBUST AND WITHSTAND ALL KINDS OF HANDLING QUITE WELL, WHILE OTHERS ARE FRAGILE AND WHEN THEY "BREAK"

OR DEGRADE MOLECULARLY, THEY BECOME QUITE toxic to your body. A little knowledge goes a long way in protecting yourself from unnecessary inflammation.

Manmade fats require the most vigilance—they are the kind that are only achieved through tremendous processing. What we've been conditioned to call "vegetable oils" since the 1950s are not as innocent as they sound. These oils, like canola, soybean, sunflower, and corn, are some of the most *unreal* foods in the modern food system. Though cheap and abundant, the inconvenient truth is that they are not vegetables at all—they are industrially processed seed oils. This means they have seriously damaging inflammatory effects on the human body, especially when heated (possibly even *more* damaging than the dreaded trans fats that have recently been banned). In fact, seed oils are so toxic, as well as so pervasive in our society, that I believe that they are the new sugar: a pressing public-health concern.

Steer clear of processed foods (including most bottled salad dressings!) and you'll avoid a lot of these troubling oils. But it's also imperative to do a clean sweep in your kitchen. Don't worry: There's never been a better time to do this oil audit, because a new wave of food producers, like Fatworks and Paleo Butter Co, are making superb quality "real fats" for cooking, inspired by older methods. Pick two or three to have on hand, or more if you love to cook! Then follow the simple guidelines that follow for safe storing and cooking.

REAL OIL VS. FAKE OIL: THE SAFETY SPECTRUM

The oil you choose, and the way you use it—frying, gentle sautéing, or using it cold and raw—does make a difference. Keep a variety on hand, and vary according to your use. Knowing the "smoke point"—the highest temperature a fat can reach before it starts to smoke and produce damaging byproducts—helps you stay in the safety zone. Remember, whatever goes *into* the fats, like GMO feed, growth hormones, and pesticides, or luscious green grass that converts to fat-soluble vitamins, ultimately goes into *you*! Fats are highly concentrated, therefore precious, foods. A value price of $3 a quart should give you serious pause.

GREEN LIGHT

BEEF TALLOW: Versatile, shelf-stable. Great for baking, sautéing, frying eggs, making stews, or (very occasionally!) deep-frying. Look for 100 percent grass-fed.

LARD: Rendered fat from pigs, able to withstand medium to high heat. Great for baking and occasional frying. Seek fully pasture-raised.

GOOSE AND DUCK FAT: Rich flavor. Try it for roasting vegetables and cooking omelets. Seek pasture-raised, supplemented with non-GMO feed if necessary.

GRASS-FED BUTTER: A nutrient-rich fat if you tolerate dairy well. Use to spread, or for medium-heat cooking (butter can burn at high heat).

GRASS-FED GHEE: Butter that has been "clarified" (heated and separated) to create oil without the milk proteins.

OXIDATION, NOT SATURATION: THE REAL HEALTH CULPRIT

We used to cook primarily using butter and lard. These robust saturated fats don't change much when heated—they are stable and dependable. But when newfangled, manmade fats were introduced in the early twentieth century, things changed. First, artificial trans fats, made by adding hydrogen to harden seed oils, were invented to make mass-processed and fast foods easier and cheaper to produce. Though we recently wised up to their damaging contribution to heart disease, diabetes, and much more, highly refined seed oils, many made from GMO plants, have now taken their place. These oils are high in the fatty acids that cause inflammation and increase the risk of multiple disease processes. They are typically processed using harsh, petroleum-based chemicals to increase their shelf life. Worst of all, they degrade when heated to release toxic compounds of all kinds, including a group of volatile and very inflammatory compounds called aldehydes. Heart disease, gastric damage, cancer, neurodegenerative diseases . . . you name it, it's linked to these compounds.

BUY WISELY, STORE SMARTLY

For plant oils, organic, unrefined, and expeller pressed are best. Since fragile plant fats degrade quickly, store them away from direct sunlight, ideally in dark bottles. Buy smaller amounts and use within three months. (Consider freezing any excess you can't use soon.)

IF YOU EAT OUT ON A DAILY BASIS, INVISIble seed oils will be part of your meals. Most non-gourmet restaurants (and all fast-food restaurants) use them, often at high heat. Avoid fried foods, and don't be shy about asking the staff how things are cooked or prepped. Your best bet is something simply prepared, without cooking oils, that you can top with good olive oil if it is available.

There's no vegetable benefit to be gained from vegetable oil.

High smoke point, equally delicious stirred into hot foods and drinks. Some brands are now lab verified to contain no milk proteins.

COCONUT OIL: A heat-safe fat that takes medium to high heat well. Has immune-boosting effects. Look for oil that is not deodorized or bleached.

PALM OIL: Another robust plant fat for medium-high heat. Caution! Only choose unrefined, sustainably sourced palm oil—since the palm oil industry can cause tremendous harm to rain forest ecologies, make sure your brand is "conflict free."

OLIVE OIL: Use raw for dressings and dips, or cook over low heat only. Buy with care: Look for genuine extra-virgin that is under eighteen months old. See howtobewell.com for how to buy real olive oil, not fake or rancid oils.

AVOCADO OIL: Neutral taste, withstands high-heat cooking. Great for a lighter-flavored mayonnaise.

FLAXSEED AND HEMP OIL: Raw use only! Use on salads, or in smoothies for a dose of fats. Keep in the fridge and use quickly.

RED LIGHT—AVOID—PROCESSED AND UNNATURAL FATS

VEGETABLE OIL: A misnomer—there are no vegetables in these bottles. Likely a mix of chemically extracted industrial seed oils, especially GMO soybeans.

MARGARINES AND SPREADS: Altered seed oils, further chemically processed to become a faux saturate. Contain proinflammatory ingredients—don't accept these sketchy substitutions!

CANOLA OIL: An extremely refined oil, created by hybridizing industrial rapeseeds. Can include (unlabeled) trans fats.

CORN OIL: Highly chemically processed, highly inflammatory, usually GMO-laced.

SAFFLOWER OIL AND SUNFLOWER OIL: Typically extracted with hexane (which is believed to be a neurotoxin), high in inflammatory fatty acids.

PEANUT OIL: Skews higher in the inflammatory fatty acids, contains lectins.

So-called "vegetable" oils are actually made from tough seeds and legumes that were originally grown for industrial use, not human consumption.

No matter what size your dinner, finish eating at least two to three hours before you go to bed.

EAT IN RHYTHM

EAT YOUR LARGEST MEAL OF THE DAY AT LUNCH, IN SYNC WITH WHEN THE SUN IS AT ITS ZENITH, AND A SMALLER MEAL AT NIGHT, AS THE SUN SINKS OUT OF SIGHT. YOUR METABOLISM—THE COLLECTIVE WORD FOR THE INNUMERABLE BIOLOGICAL PROCESSES THAT SUSTAIN LIFE—RISES THROUGHOUT THE DAY, IN TANDEM

WITH YOUR BODY TEMPERATURE. THE "CLOCK" IN your GI tract triggers hormones that set off hunger pangs and cue the liver and digestive system to get ready to process nutrients. This signaling reaches its peak at midday, preparing your body to eat its largest amount of food.

As sunset approaches, your body clock stops triggering active and productive hormones, your temperature falls, and your metabolism slows down. Your physiology winds down in sync with the day. This means your digestive system is not as ready for a large meal at night, which is why many people find that digestion and elimination, as well as sleep, are more satisfying with substantial lunches and lighter (sometimes soup-based) dinners. Experiment

with a light dinner and see how you feel the next morning. Though you might not know it consciously, your body prefers this gentler state: Since it does not need many calories for sleep, adding excess fuel late at night can generate excessive free radicals that damage tissues, promote aging, and even contribute to chronic disease. The closer you are to a "fasted," or non-digesting, state overnight, the better it is for your health.

The takeaway: No matter what size your dinner, finish eating at least two to three hours before you go to bed. That way, your body can prioritize recovery and rebuilding during sleep instead of laboring to digest.

JUICE SMART,
GO GREEN

IT'S A GREAT IDEA TO MASTER A JUICING HABIT. DONE right, it can give your body an infusion of phytochemicals, micronutrients, and electrolytes in an easily absorbable form, making juice a good pick-me-up and a gentle way to get nutrition when you want to rest your digestion.

But juicing done wrong can be a disaster, spiking blood sugar and triggering the kind of sugar overload that sends your body into metabolic chaos. Juicing fruits, as well as higher-carbohydrate vegetables like carrots or beets, delivers a rush of fructose (see page 28) in liquid form, without any of the fiber. When you eat the *whole* apple, orange, or ruby-red beet, it's the fiber that slows the sugar's entry into your cells so you can metabolize them more slowly and safely. Fruity juices can be so high in sugars—I once counted 38 grams at a local juice joint!—that drinking them is like drinking soda, without the bubbles. (Always check the sugar content of any bottled or store-made juice you order—even if it's green in color.)

If you like juicing, make it a tool you use frequently. But use it as a supplement to an already vegetable-rich diet, not a substitution for eating vegetables. Once again I stress sticking to low-carbohydrate vegetables, principally the green and white kinds like hydrating cucumbers, mineral-rich celery, and leafy greens like spinach, chard, and small amounts of kale (unless you have thyroid issues) and dandelion. You can also include roots with detoxifying and immunity-boosting benefits like burdock and ginger, and herbs like parsley and cilantro—but use zero fruit, save for lime or lemon or maybe a little tart green apple.

The resulting drinks may not seem perfectly palatable—at first—because they don't hit the sweet-and-fruity flavor profile your taste buds expect. But follow the guidelines that follow and you will soon find your groove. And know that the benefits of this habit go well beyond the ingestion of nutrients. Drinking green juice often paves the way for

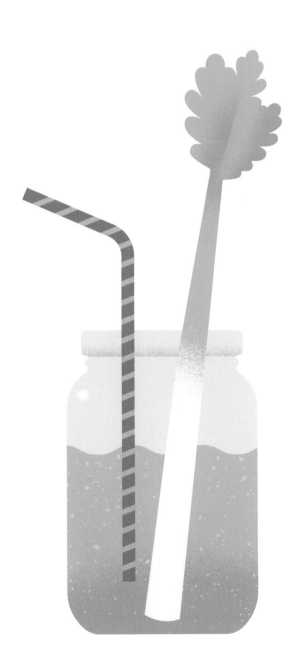

an upgraded diet. It contributes to a rewiring of eating patterns: Consuming vegetables galore shifts your palate and reshapes your desires. Soon you'll find that fresh, whole ingredients become the foods your body craves.

GOING GREENER: A GRADUAL TRANSITION

Make green juices your go-to by training your palate to like the taste of green. Rather than leaping into the greenest shade and deciding you just don't like it at all, ease your way in more slowly.

STEP 1 Commit to nixing the supersweet ingredients like fruit, and keep sugary vegetables like beets to just one part of a green-filled blend (and only occasionally, not every day).

STEP 2 Enjoy mildly green juices that use celery and cucumber along with accents like lemon and ginger. Handfuls of spinach and romaine can boost nutrition without adding too much strong flavor. A small amount of tart green apple works here to give a touch of sweetness.

STEP 3 Gradually increase the darker greens in your mix (taking out your apple "crutch"). The bitter tastes of chard and kale signal that liver-supporting phytochemicals are at work.

STEP 4 Once dark-green juice becomes your new normal, begin to experiment with intense ingredients that broaden the health benefits and the flavor profile. Try cilantro and burdock root for detoxification, anticancer collards, blood-boosting wheatgrass shots, and liver-protective dandelion.

Note: If your produce is not organic, peel before juicing.

Fruity juices can be so high in sugars that drinking them is like drinking soda, without the bubbles.

◀◀

USE SPICE AS
DAILY MEDICINE

SPICES ARE YOUR ALLIES IN THE PROJECT OF STICKING TO HEALTHY HOME COOKING. THEY HELP YOU GET INFINITE COMBINATIONS OF TASTY MEALS FROM BASIC WHOLE FOODS (ROAST CHICKEN, GRILLED FISH, STIR-FRIED VEGETABLES, AND MORE), AND THEY KEEP YOUR SENSES EXCITED. IN MANY AMERICAN KITCHENS, SPICES

LOITER, BARELY USED, IN KITCHEN CUPBOARDS, WHICH is a mistake, because when meals are overly bland, heavily flavored processed foods become even more craveable! Furthermore, spices can act as medicine: Many cuisines worldwide use them liberally to aid digestion and nutrient absorption. Today, science is showing us that many everyday spices, like cinnamon, cloves, turmeric, and ginger are highly concentrated antioxidant powerhouses that also contain antiviral, antibacterial, antifungal, and anticancer components. Using them liberally throughout the day is a simple way to infuse more protective benefits into your diet.

I've watched chefs play with spices as freely as kids play with paint colors—when making dinner in a new kitchen, their very first move is to check out the spice cabinet. My longtime friend, master chef David Bouley, has a food-as-pharmacy philosophy and deploys spices fearlessly for healing and pleasure. At his workshops he teaches a nifty trick for getting spices out of the bottle and into food: infusing them into oils for dressings, drizzling, and sautéing. "The oil protects the spice from oxidation, preserving and rounding out its fullest flavor," he says. While he employs several professional techniques to make the oils (different spices release their beneficial "terpenes" at different temperatures), the following oil can easily be made at home with a basic infusing technique. Combine your spice with a high-quality oil, and you will have two good foods in one.

DAVID BOULEY'S ANTI-INFLAMMATORY TURMERIC OIL

HOW TO BE WELL EXPERT

Many people know that curcumin, the active component in turmeric, is a powerful anti-inflammatory with a host of protective qualities (such as promoting a healthy response from gut flora, tonifying the liver, boosting immunity, protecting against dementia, and more). But few of us feel confident about how to use it. This oil makes turmeric an everyday accent, and David advises to experiment with it: It can be used for drizzling on vegetables (I love stirring it into carrot soup), topping organic popcorn that's been popped in heat-tolerant coconut oil or lard, whisking into salad dressings, or topping zoodles or grain-free pasta. A grind of black pepper helps activate the turmeric's healing power, and some shavings of good Parmesan, if you eat dairy, will make your seven-minute meal feel totally gourmet.

In his chef's kitchen, David uses 1 cup ground turmeric to 30 tablespoons of oil, which is a blend of equal parts avocado, grapeseed, and extra-virgin olive oil. To customize this for home use, simply blend one part ground turmeric with two parts oil (or oils) of choice, experimenting with the different types of oil to see which you prefer.

1. FILL A GLASS BOTTLE OR JAR with the oil and turmeric.

2. COVER AND LET SIT away from light for 2 weeks before use.

You can also infuse oils with ginger, garlic, or vanilla, which help with joint inflammation, candida overgrowth, and digestive function.

8 SPICE AND HERB MUST-HAVES

David Bouley works with more than 1,900 spices, but you don't need to build a spice bazaar. Commit to using just two or three of these easy-to-find culinary accents at first. Then slowly build up your repertoire, and soon you will have a vibrant food culture in your home!

1. **ONE OR MORE ANTI-INFLAMMATORY SPICES** like turmeric (this may be in a curry mix), fresh ginger, or garlic—try adding turmeric and ginger to smoothies

2. **CAYENNE PEPPER,** to boost the immune system— add a pinch to hot chocolate

3. **VANILLA BEANS, PASTE, OR PURE EXTRACT** to increase the perception of sweetness in foods, reducing the need for sugar

4. **CINNAMON,** for stabilizing blood sugar—use it in homemade chai tea with cardamom and ginger. Grind it yourself from sticks for maximum freshness.

5. **TARRAGON,** for deep French bistro flavor—try it on chicken and in lentil soup

6. **SESAME,** to add protein and magnesium—sprinkle it on top of proteins or vegetables

7. **PARSLEY AND CILANTRO** (fresh or dried), to impart a lively, fresh taste as well as vitamins and minerals. Scatter in salads, soups, and on proteins of all kinds, experimenting with flavor (cilantro is especially good with Mexican, Indian, and Southeast Asian dishes).

8. **MUSHROOMS** (like dried shiitake), for anti-disease and antibacterial properties—add them to broths and soups

>>
Combine your spice with a high-quality oil, and you will have two good foods in one.
<<

BECOME A **FAT-BURNER**

THE BIG NEWS IN NUTRITION-AS-MEDICINE IS KETOGENIC EATING. IT TAKES THE LOW-CARB DIET (PAGE 85) ONE STEP FURTHER. KETOGENIC EATING INVOLVES FOLLOWING A CUSTOMIZED LOW-CARB, MODERATE-PROTEIN, HIGH-FAT DIET IN ORDER TO SWITCH ON A METABOLIC STATE IN WHICH THE BODY USES THE ENERGY FROM FAT

(KETONES AND FATTY ACIDS) TO POWER ITS NEEDS instead of the energy from starches and sugars (glucose). This diet has to be maintained pretty rigorously (no sudden deviations like a dessert here or sugary latte there!), but the result is that after a few weeks of adaptation, the body uses a new energy pathway: It burns fat for energy, first the quality fat you consume in your diet, and then the fat stored on your body.

Until recently, the protocol was mainly known for its ability to reduce or prevent seizures in those with epilepsy, but today we're discovering that it can have major benefits for those with what are largely seen as "lifestyle" diseases (i.e., relating primarily to insulin-disrupting, inflammatory diets). Weight problems, type 2 diabetes and metabolic syndrome, cardiovascular disease, polycystic ovary syndrome, irritable bowel syndrome, GERD and heartburn, and nonalcoholic fatty liver disease are just some of the conditions that see benefits from ketogenic eating. Emerging evidence suggests benefits for a host of neurological conditions as well. Though at first it requires a will of steel to commit to this unwavering way of eating, advocates report that the benefits soon establish the habit—and

without the dangers and side effects of drugs! Those who implement a ketogenic diet also report that they function with better mental clarity, feel less hunger throughout the day, and see improved blood work markers for insulin sensitivity and blood sugars.

If weight loss is proving difficult or you have any of the conditions mentioned above, start on a low-carb diet and then consider graduating to a well-formulated ketogenic eating plan for three months to see how it works for you. I recommend working with your doctor, especially if you have serious health issues, and monitoring your blood sugar and ketone levels if you are starting from a health-compromised position. (The Nova Max monitor measures both sugars and ketones). Whatever your motivation for trying this protocol, remember to get your proteins and your fats from the best-quality sources you can.

Tip: To take a deep dive into the philosophy, protocols, and practices of a ketogenic diet, check out the books *Primal Fat Burner* by Nora Gedgaudas, CNS, NTP, BCHN, and *Keto Clarity* by Jimmy Moore with Eric Westman, MD.

A ketogenic diet shifts your metabolism from a carbohydrate-burning machine to a fat-burning one.

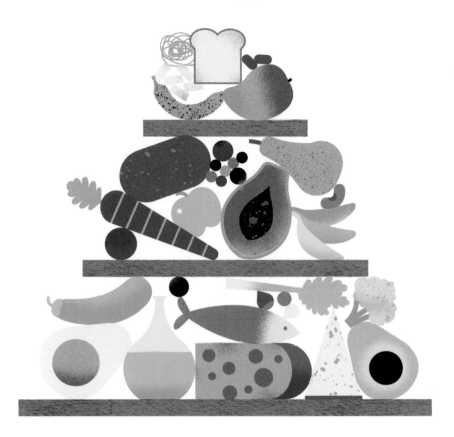

CUSTOMIZE YOUR CARBS:

CUSTOMIZE YOUR CARBS:
DISCOVER IF "HEALTHY" CARBS ARE HELPING OR HURTING YOU

CARBOHYDRATE TOLERANCE IS A GRAY AREA. THE AMOUNT OF CARBOHYDRATES THAT WORKS FOR ONE PERSON'S METABOLISM DOESN'T ALWAYS SERVE ANOTHER'S. IN THE PAST DECADE I'VE SEEN A GROWING NUMBER OF PATIENTS WHO HAVE LIMITED SUGARY FOODS AND SWAPPED OUT REFINED CARBOHYDRATES FOR

WHOLE-GRAIN PRODUCTS, SWEET POTATOES, AND fresh fruit for years. Yet they are overweight or have surges of fatigue, foggy-headedness, or cravings. Sometimes they don't carry any extra pounds but have worryingly high levels of blood sugar. It's not unusual for these issues to come on late in life; their response to a diet they used to do well on has suddenly shifted.

Why this happens is a topic of robust debate in nutritional circles. It's likely a combination of factors: a genetic predisposition combined with a sedentary, stressful, and sleep-deprived lifestyle; decades of processed foods and medications that have altered the microbiome; or even (unfortunately) overconsuming the healthy-seeming multigrain breads, bananas, and beans, which all turn to sugar in the blood. All this can lower your personal "set point" for tolerating carbohydrates, so that your blood sugars don't fall back to normal within two hours of eating like they should. Instead, they stay elevated, going beyond what the cells can handle, and eventually this triggers chains of effects that lead to insulin resistance, the precursor to high blood pressure, heart disease, diabetes, obesity, possibly Alzheimer's disease, and even some cancers. The 2017 National Diabetes Statistics report found that an estimated 50 percent of Americans have either diabetes or prediabetes—and that many are unaware of this fact. Taking your blood sugar seriously is nothing to sneeze at.

When carb intolerance is at play, your body is telling you to get stricter with your intake. To follow a low-carb diet, nix all sugars and reduce complex carbs dramatically, replacing them with plenty of nonstarchy vegetables and generous amounts of fat. In addition, take sleep seriously, work on repairing the gut (page 174), and increase the amount of movement you do. The low-carb diet, along with these other fundamental improvements, can often help restore order where there was previously metabolic chaos. To catalyze real metabolic change in cases of significant weight gain or diabetes, it may be warranted to take the low-carb approach to its ultimate extreme: the ketogenic protocol (page 84).

There is another, more accurate way to learn your personal carb set point. Use a glucose monitor to measure the impact of a range of carbohydrate-rich foods on your blood sugar. Twice after eating, at the one-hour and two-hour mark, you can get snapshots of how your body metabolizes starches like grains, beans, and potatoes.

If this level of detective work speaks to you, try the protocol outlined in Robb Wolf's book *Wired to Eat*. His program of dietary change, basic blood work, and a seven-day carb test can help you zero in on your set point and your level of insulin resistance.

SO I AM CARB INTOLERANT: NOW WHAT?

Take heart! Healthy low-carb diets can improve blood pressure and help you lose weight, have fewer sugar cravings, and feel less driven by hunger. Skin and digestion often improve, as well as triglycerides (a form of blood lipids) and blood sugar and insulin markers.

Follow all the advice in this section—then tweak your diet slightly using the suggestions that follow:

• **NO SUGARS OR REFINED CARBOHYDRATES.**

• **INCREASE THE AMOUNT OF LEAFY AND CRUCIFEROUS VEGETABLES** at each meal, and dramatically or completely decrease complex carbs like starchy vegetables; grains, beans, and legumes; and "pseudo grains" like quinoa and buckwheat. Maximum two or three portions of these complex carbs per week.

• **BE MORE GENEROUS THAN YOU THINK YOU SHOULD BE WITH "GOOD" FATS** like avocados and EVOO.

• **LIMIT DAIRY** (it's high in carbs).

• **LOW-SUGAR FRESH OR FROZEN FRUIT ONLY:** fresh berries, citrus fruits, green apples, maximum two or three times a week.

• **GO VERY LIGHT ON THE ALCOHOL,** and if you do drink, go for the lowest-carb options. Pure spirits like whiskey, vodka, and tequila are carb-free, and dry wine is better than beer. Avoid sweet drinks and mixers, which may contain a lot of sugar.

• **PAY ATTENTION TO THE EFFECTS OF STARCHY FOODS** when you do eat them. Your tolerance can rise and fall depending on how much you exercised, how well you slept, how stressed you are, and so on. There's nothing a doctor can give you that is more valuable than this personal awareness.

If you find that you handle whole-food complex carbs quite well, I still advise that you keep them to a reasonable amount, picking from the low- and medium-count foods described above. If you are using carb-counting devices, know this: Conventional dietary recommendations suggest a limit of 225 grams per day. That's too high: Stay under 150 grams a day maximum, and preferably under 100 grams.

AM I CARBOHYDRATE INTOLERANT? TAKE THE QUIZ

START BY ANSWERING THESE QUESTIONS.

1. Are you overweight?
2. Do you feel fatigued much of the time, especially after eating a carb-heavy meal?
3. Do you lead a largely sedentary life?
4. Do you feel like your appetite is out of control?
5. Do you frequently crave sweets or starchy foods like bread, pasta, potatoes, or beans?
6. Do you feel light-headed and dizzy when you get hungry?
7. Is your blood sugar in the upper ranges of "normal" or beyond?
8. Are you struggling with brain fog, anxiety, depression, skin problems, joint pain, aching muscles, hormonal issues, and/or sleep problems?

OPTIONAL: If you've had blood work done recently, look at your hemoglobin A1c levels. This provides a snapshot into your average blood sugar levels over the last three months. Has your diet been clear of sugary foods, yet the number is still above 5.5?

If you answered yes to one or more questions, try fourteen days of cutting out of your diet all grains, legumes (beans and peas), starchy vegetables (carrots, corn, potatoes, squash, sweet potatoes, yams), and fruit. (In case it's not obvious, sugary foods, natural sweeteners like honey, maple syrup, and agave, and most packaged drinks should be removed completely.) After day 14, revisit questions 2, 5, 6, and 8. If you have experienced a marked change in your symptoms, you may have discovered your own carbohydrate intolerance.

Carbohydrate intolerance means you are eating more carbs than your system can process efficiently.

EAT DINNER EARLIER AND BREAKFAST LATER:
INTERMITTENT FASTING

FOR MILLENNIA, HUMANS FEASTED AND FASTED IN REGULAR CYCLES, BY NECESSITY. (ANIMAL HUNTS DIDN'T DELIVER MEALS AT REGULAR FOUR-HOUR INTERVALS!) TODAY, WE DO THE OPPOSITE, EATING MORE OR LESS IN A CONTINUUM, FAR FROM OUR ANCESTRAL NORM OF PERIODS OF FOOD-FREE, METABOLIC "DOWNTIME,"

WHICH MAY BE ONE CAUSE OF THE WEIGHT GAIN AND metabolic disruption that have become so common. Introducing deliberate periods of extended fasting to mimic these evolutionary norms can get your body back to metabolic regulation when it is out of balance. It's a tool you can try if you're struggling to lose weight or keep your blood sugars and insulin levels in healthy range. You can also use it proactively to maintain good health: Fasting initiates cellular repair processes like autophagy, which removes waste material from cells and helps dampen inflammation, slows down aging, and optimizes mitochondrial function, giving you greater protection against disease.

WHAT IT IS:

Intermittent fasting is a protocol of periodically waiting about sixteen hours between meals, typically between your last meal of one day and your first meal of the next. This lets your body enter a prolonged "fasting state" and signals your metabolism to burn fat that is stored on the body. It also allows your body to experience a longer-than-normal period of low insulin in the blood. This tells your body to burn energy and keep insulin low, which is a powerful reset and the opposite of what happens with a constant stream of food.

Intermittent fasting is not a promise of sudden weight loss; it's about reeducating the hormones to return to more regulated functioning as part of a longer-term weight loss protocol. Done consistently, it can help blood glucose, blood pressure, and liver function markers to nor-

malize. Some people use IF weekly as a preventive tool against diseases of modern civilization like heart disease, stroke, cancer, fatty liver, polycystic ovarian syndrome, and Alzheimer's disease. Others use a more intensified version of IF to manage and mitigate diseases like type 2 diabetes and obesity. Intermittent fasting experts like Dr. Jason Fung believe that the protocol can also improve your relationship to food by empowering you with a tool to balance out occasional indulgences and giving new clarity about what "hunger" actually is.

HOW TO DO IT:

Simply wait about sixteen hours between your last meal of day one and your first meal of day two. If you finish dinner at 8:00 p.m., your next meal—the time you "break the fast"—will be at or around 12:00 p.m. the following day. If you have dinner at 5:00 p.m., your next meal will be around 9:00 a.m.

HOW OFTEN TO FAST:

One or two days per week for basic preventive measures.

If experimenting with IF feels too extreme, focus instead on the golden rule of good digestion: Always leave at least twelve hours between dinner and breakfast to let your body direct energy toward healing and detoxifying overnight.

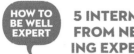

5 INTERMITTENT FASTING TIPS FROM NEPHROLOGIST AND FASTING EXPERT JASON FUNG, MD

1. **AS WITH ANY NEW SKILL, THE FIRST FEW TIMES FASTING ARE ALWAYS DIFFICULT.** Give your body a month to get used to it. While annoying side effects like constipation, cramps, and headaches can occur during fasting, there are simple tips than can help that I outline in my books. Many of these side effects go away as your body gets used to fasting.

2. **STAY BUSY, AS IT KEEPS YOUR MIND OFF FOOD.** Fasting during a busy day at work is often easiest.

3. **YOU WILL GET HUNGRY,** especially at your accustomed meal times, but it will pass. Hunger does not build continuously but passes like a wave. Ignore it, and your hunger will fade.

4. **STICKING TO A LOW-CARBOHYDRATE, HIGH-FAT DIET** before fasting often makes it easier.

5. **DO ALL YOUR USUAL ACTIVITIES.** Continue your usual exercise routine. Your body will get all the energy it requires from your body fat.

(IF is not indicated for pregnant or breastfeeding women, children under 18, or the malnourished or underweight [BMI<20]. If you are taking medication, consult your physician.)

To learn more about intermittent fasting, read Dr. Fung's books *The Obesity Code* and *The Complete Guide to Fasting*.

Intermittent fasting is a tool you can try if you're struggling to lose weight or keep your blood sugars and insulin levels in healthy range. You can also use it proactively to maintain good health.

DETECT YOUR FOOD
SENSITIVITIES

IF YOU FEEL IN ANY WAY LESS THAN OPTIMAL—AND THE PARAMETERS ARE WIDE HERE AND INCLUDE ANY CHRONIC PROBLEM FROM DIGESTIVE DISTRESS, BLOATING AND WEIGHT GAIN, BRAIN FOG AND HEADACHES, FATIGUE, SKIN ISSUES, JOINT PAIN, DEPRESSION, AND MORE—USE AN ELIMINATION DIET TO FIGURE OUT IF SOME

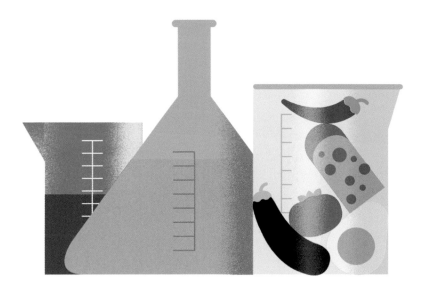

OF THE FUNDAMENTAL FOODS IN YOUR DIET ARE a cause. Often, a food can have caused invisible inflammation for years, without you even knowing. Food sensitivity wasn't always the big issue it is today, making it hard to deny that something has changed in the ways food is produced and the compromised state of our gut microbiome, which causes the gut wall to become damaged. An increasing number of foods are causing sensitivities in my patients; grains and beans are some of the newest culprits, probably due to lectins (see page 37).

While any dietary changes require effort and willpower, the good news is that this common-sense protocol costs nothing, requires no lab tests or supervision, and often ignites a new self-awareness and a commitment to using food wisely. The *great* news is that detecting a "trigger food"—something that triggers uncomfortable symptoms—and then eliminating it from your diet can help you start to feel better in ten days to two weeks (however, if it's part of a more complex autoimmune disease, the process may take several months). Here's how to follow a standard elimination diet for at least two weeks.

STEP 1 Download the Food Sensitivity Questionnaire from howtobewell.com to get an initial gauge of your symptoms.

STEP 2 Choose to do a basic protocol, which targets the main trigger foods: gluten, dairy, corn, and soy. Or choose the more complete protocol, which includes secondary offenders: eggs, nightshades (tomatoes, bell peppers, white potatoes, and eggplant, all of which can cause inflammation and joint pain), grains, legumes, and peanuts. Many people do a "clean sweep" and remove all of these foods, which is what I recommend in my Be Well Cleanse (a complete cleanse program that includes nutrients and supplements, which also help address microbiome imbalance and the detoxification process). But it's fine to keep it simple: Start with the basic protocol, and then test the complete-protocol foods if symptoms have not resolved.

STEP 3 For two weeks, eliminate all the foods you want to test. Use the information in this section to get ideas for healthy whole-food meals that keep you nourished. Try not to load up your plate with packaged "free-from" foods (processed foods marked "gluten-free," "dairy-free," "egg-free," etc.). Use the resources at howtobewell.com for more ideas.

STEP 4 When the two weeks are up, reintroduce *one* of the "excluded" foods back into your diet every two to three days, to check your reaction to that food. On each reintroduction day, eat at least one to two portions of that food, then for the next 24 to 48 hours, refer to the Food Sensitivity Questionnaire and make a note of any symptoms you experience. Typically, after a period of elimination, you will experience a more pronounced reaction to a trigger food than usual, because when you eat a food daily, its aggravating effect can be harder to feel. A pronounced reaction is a clear clue that the food is aggravating you and should be eliminated for good.

In the reintroduction phase, be careful not to eat foods like pizza, which includes three excluded foods (dairy, gluten, tomato). If you have a reaction, you won't know what caused it.

STEP 5 If the elimination diet does not deliver the clues you are seeking, turn to "What to Do When . . ." on page 245 for more guidance on FODMAPs and removing other commonly aggravating foods.

WHERE BLOOD TESTS FIT IN

I tend to favor simple self-evaluations like the elimination diet over laboratory testing because I have seen too many inconclusive results over my career. However, newer labs like Cyrex Labs are changing the game by offering state-of-the-art food sensitivity tests that can even determine which tissue groups are being affected by inflammatory reactions. These tests can be a helpful resource if you are not getting satisfactory answers from the elimination diet, but they are expensive and not available everywhere.

WIN FOOD FREEDOM!
A DOCTOR'S MANIFESTO

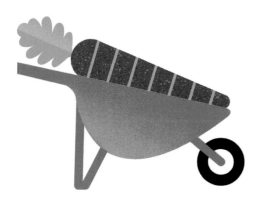

EAT REAL, WHOLE FOODS.

THE LESS ALTERED AND MANIPULATED THE BETTER.

READ INGREDIENTS RELIGIOUSLY.

YOU WILL TRAIN YOURSELF TO ASSESS FOODS WITH A SINGLE, SPEEDY GLANCE.

WAKE UP!

OUR PALATES HAVE BEEN SHAPED BY INDUSTRY AGENDAS AND GOVERNMENT GUIDELINES, NOT TRUE METABOLIC AND NUTRITIONAL NEEDS.

DON'T COUNT CALORIES.

FOCUS MORE ON QUALITY, STRESS LESS ABOUT QUANTITY, AND DISCOVER WHAT IRRITATES AND INFLAMES YOUR BODY.

BUY VEGETABLES LIKE YOUR LIFE DEPENDS ON IT.

RAW, STEAMED, ROASTED, SPROUTED. TRY TO HAVE THEM AT EVERY MEAL.

CLEAN FOOD IS YOUR FUNDA-MENTAL RIGHT.

TOXINS AND CHEMICALS MAY HAVE BECOME THE NORM—BUT YOU DON'T NEED TO ACCEPT THEM.

BUY AN APRON . . . BUT LOWER THE BAR.

NOT EVERY MEAL YOU MAKE HAS TO BE *TOP CHEF*-PERFECT.

QUESTION YOUR BELIEFS.

THINK THAT HEALTHY FOOD COSTS MORE? BUY BULK INGREDIENTS, PREP YOUR MEALS AT HOME—THEN THINK AGAIN.

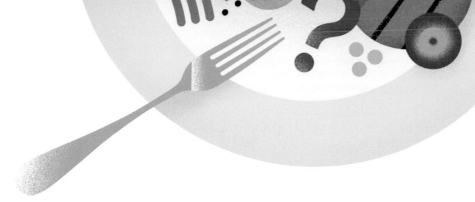

EAT DINNER EARLIER AND (OCCASIONALLY) EAT BREAKFAST LATER.

REST YOUR DIGESTION. IT WILL THANK YOU.

PAY THE FARMER NOW, NOT THE PHARMACIST (OR DOCTOR) LATER.

FRESH GOOD FOOD TODAY COSTS LESS THAN MEDICAL BILLS LATER. (AND IT'S A LOT MORE FUN.)

BE SKEPTICAL.

ESPECIALLY OF FOODS THAT ARE TOO GOOD TO BE TRUE. COOL LOGOS CAN'T MASK CRAPPY INGREDIENTS.

WALK YOUR OWN PATH.

EVEN IF THE PEOPLE YOU LIVE WITH AND WORK WITH AREN'T ON IT . . .

. . . BUT CHOW DOWN WITH OTHERS!

COOKING AND EATING TOGETHER FEEDS BODY, MIND, AND SOUL.

AND ALWAYS REMEMBER, THE FOODS THAT ARE BEST FOR YOU DO NOT NEED A LABEL, BOX, OR BAG.

THEY COME THE WAY NATURE INTENDED: NAKED.

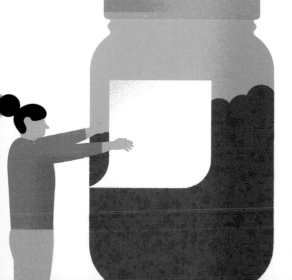
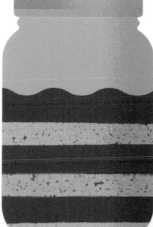
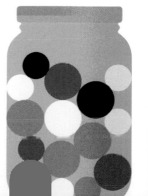
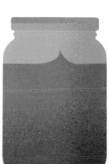

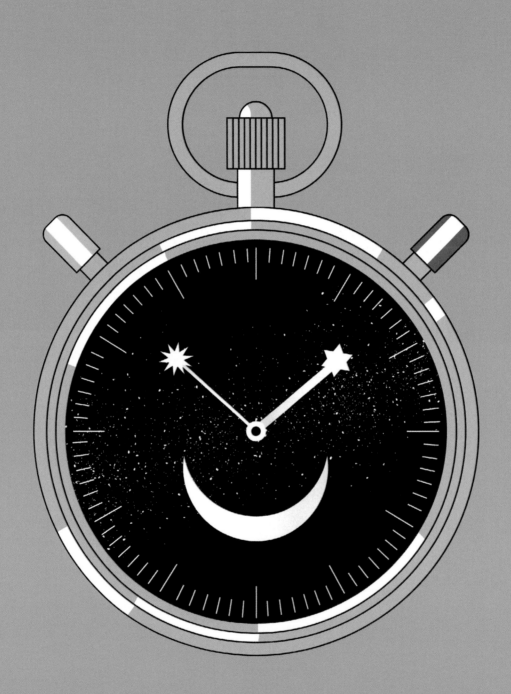

SLEEP

"TELL ME HOW TO SLEEP!" IS ONE OF THE MOST common refrains in my practice. We've never, as a population, been as sleep-deprived and sleep-deranged as today. This takes a serious toll, because sleep is a cornerstone of wellness: It's essential for focused mental performance, a stable mood, a strong immune system, a healthy stress response, proper cellular repair, and a healthy metabolism. It's when your body does much of its disease-fighting maintenance work.

Too often, when sleep is off track, the temptation is to paper over the cracks with nocturnal TV watching, wine, medication, and other unnatural sleep aids. But these crutches—which sometimes have side effects—won't help you sleep better long-term, and they can stop you from looking deeper for the cause. When your sleep goes awry, it's a clue that something about your lifestyle is asking to be adjusted, or that something else in your body needs attention. The actions and habits in this ring will help you make those adjustments and learn more about how you, and your sleep tendencies, tick. The tricky thing about sleep is that what works for one person does not always work for the next, but nobody gets away from the obvious: One root cause of nighttime sleep problems is daytime stress.

If you frequently shortchange yourself on sleep, it might be time to reevaluate. Chronic poor sleep will play itself out in myriad negative ways because snooze is your key rhythm, the master conductor that keeps *all* your body's rhythms humming in tune.

WHY BETTER SLEEP MATTERS, **OR 12 REASONS TO PRIORITIZE SLEEP TONIGHT**

1 Lack of sleep can make you fatter, biologically older, and more at risk for heart disease and diabetes.

2 70 percent of Americans get insufficient sleep today.

3 We typically sleep two hours less than we did four decades ago. Now we are learning that losing two hours of sleep causes inflammatory markers to appear. (You also lose out on the natural increase in cancer-fighting molecules in the body; these have been measured to rise tenfold during sleep, then fall again on waking.)

4 Don't sacrifice sleep to get to the gym. Sleep is primary. Exercise is secondary.

5 Eight hours is best (though individual needs vary).

6 Surrender to bed! When you're tired, say, "I'm tired" and act accordingly.

7 Unwind your buzzing brain every day. A state of hyperarousal is the enemy of sleep.

8 Productivity and positivity surge with good sleep. Depression diminishes. Do your state of mind a favor and prioritize slumber.

9 Skimp on sleep, and fight-or-flight reactions to everyday challenges will increase. The result is a body and mind that is wired for stress.

10 Did you know that healthy people start to express diabetic-like symptoms after chronic poor sleep?

11 Tempted to stay up late sexing up your social media profile? Turn off the light: Z's repair wear and tear and keep your body—and your looks—youthful!

12 Fall asleep within thirty minutes and rarely toss and turn for more than fifteen minutes during the night? Relax! You're "on track" with your sleep.

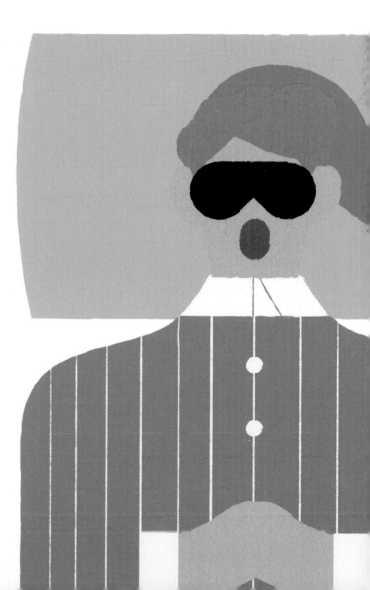

RESET YOUR BODY CLOCK

GOOD SLEEP IS A RESULT OF A DANCE BETWEEN QUANTITY (GETTING ENOUGH), QUALITY (ENSURING PHASES OF DEEP SLEEP OCCUR), AND TIMING (DOING IT IN SYNC WITH YOUR NATURAL BODY CLOCK). IT'S THE LATTER FACTOR THAT MOST TYPICALLY GETS OVERLOOKED. IN OUR WORLD OF PERSISTENT CONNECTIVITY, GLOBAL

TRAVEL, AND ON-DEMAND EVERYTHING, IT CAN FEEL baffling that there are some fundamental biological laws of timing that are bigger than you and that you can't out-think or outmaneuver.

These laws are governed by your circadian rhythm: the dominant internal clock that signals your body when to sleep, when to wake up, and when to eat. Your sleep-wake cycle is influenced by several external factors, including changes in temperature and crossing time zones (which is why jet lag throws your sleeping and eating off kilter). The primary factor that influences it, however, is exposure to regular rhythms of light and dark over 24-hour cycles. Your body, quite simply, is set up to entrain itself to the rhythm of the world you live in: to sleep when it's dark, and to be wakeful when it's light.

To get technical about it, there is a "master clock" in your brain's hypothalamus called the suprachiasmatic nucleus (SCN). It receives information from cells in the eye about the duration and brightness of light through-out the day. The SCN then sends signals to all sorts of peripheral clocks in other parts of the body—e.g., ones that trigger digestive processes in the gut and immune system function—which is one reason why, when your exposure to light and dark gets out of rhythm, so many other processes in the body can be negatively affected. There is a state of rhythmic discord and you not only have poor sleep, you feel like you are constantly swim-ming upstream.

In order to sync your sleep with darkness, the hypothala-mus signals the pineal gland to make melatonin as lights dim and dusk falls. Melatonin is your onboard sleep aid, a hormone that exists to make you sleepy and, ideally, cue you to wind down and head to bed. (It also has powerful antioxidant properties—you *need* melatonin to flow prop-erly in your 24-hour cycle to protect you from premature aging, mental fogginess, a slowing metabolism, and more. Studies suggest it even protects you against cancer.) As melatonin rises, the alertness-promoting hormone cortisol dips to a low point, turning down your activity levels. Once it is fully dark, the pineal gland rhythmically secretes melatonin with the aim of keeping you asleep so that repair and restoration can occur. Then, as dawn begins to break, the light-sensor cells detect light from the sun, melatonin secretion stops, and cortisol begins rising in order to get you ready for action.

However, if the receptor cells in the eye detect artificial light from light bulbs or devices—and they can detect this through *closed eyelids even when you are sleeping*—the ultrasensitive cells of the SCN signal the pineal gland to suppress that melatonin stream. What follows is sleep dis-ruption (and a loss of that essential health-giving stream of melatonin). So imagine what happens in today's envi-ronment, in which so many laws are turned on their head (it has been dubbed an era of "invisible incoordination"). You are bathed in bright lights at night and eat meals at odd hours. You likely don't get enough natural light during the day and, quite possibly, your bedtime is inconsistent. These all conspire to push you out of sync with nature's cadences, which sets you up for sleeping problems. If the rhythmic secretions of melatonin and cortisol get chronically out of whack, it can affect you throughout the 24-hour cycle, making you sleepless in the middle of the night or needing to nap midday. If this is combined with stress, poor diet, and chaotic meal timing, health issues affecting everything from the hormones to the heart to the brain and more can begin to manifest.

YOUR NIGHTLY SLEEP FOLLOWS A RHYTHM OF ITS OWN. AS YOU SLEEP, YOU CYCLE THROUGH four stages, ideally four or five times each night. Science is now cracking the code about how this pattern of repetitive cycles is key to the functions of sleep. Because each stage has its own role in the biology of sleep, you get more from your slumber if it is uninterrupted. That said, you don't progress in a linear fashion through the cycle—it actually goes 1, 2, 3, 4, 3, 2, 1, REM (rapid eye movement).

STAGE 1 You drift into light sleep. Your muscles quiet down, your eyes move slowly, and you can be easily woken by distractions and noise.

STAGE 2 You are still in light sleep, but now your brain waves slow down. Your body temperature and heart rate decrease as you prepare to enter deep sleep.

STAGE 3 This is the beginning of deep sleep, also known as slow-wave or delta sleep. Brain waves slow further, with only occasional faster bursts. The body begins to release a surge of growth hormone, which helps to rebuild damaged cells. Surges of energy have been measured during this time—during deep sleep, the body seems to store energy for the next day.

STAGE 4 The brain almost exclusively produces slow delta waves. Muscle activity ceases. It is difficult to wake someone from this deep slumber.

REM In rapid eye movement sleep, your dreams are more vivid—your brain is as active as when it is awake. Your eyes move in quick, random movements and your muscles are temporarily paralyzed. The REM portion of the cycle lengthens as the night progresses. Wake up during this part of deep sleep and you will feel groggy and disoriented. Get disrupted too many times in the night—by a sudden noise or snoring partner—and you will miss out on dream time, hindering your brain's ability to filter through daily events and make cognitive connections. This lack of processing time is said to be linked to depression.

How to protect yourself from exhaustion? Respect the rhythms of nature, and time your sleep to synchronize with them:

First, remember you are a microcosm of the macrocosm, held in place by a larger rhythm of light and day that exists to keep you well.

Second, make one commitment: Help your body find its routine by going to bed at the same time each night — ideally around 10:00 p.m. and definitely before 11:00 p.m. — and getting up at the same time each morning (seven to eight hours later). When you push past the body's natural wind-down cues, you often get a second wind of cortisol-induced energy, which jacks you up and makes it hard to find sleep when you try later. You become tired, but wired.

Third, avoid "social jet lag" if you can. That happens when you throw off your rhythms by staying up extra late on the weekends and then forcing yourself to revert to early rising for Monday morning. The more you can stay on rhythm all week, the easier it will be to catch and ride your natural sleep wave each night.

Not everyone's circadian rhythm is the same. Some people are wired to be night owls while others are more naturally larks—early to bed, early to rise. (In technical terms, this is called being a late chronotype or an early chronotype.) Whichever type you are, the melatonin-sleepy cue should always be your signal to get into bed.

To wind the clock back on your bedtime: For several nights in a row, turn in ten minutes earlier than you normally would, until you achieve your desired earlier time. To sync your body clock to nature's master clock through exposure to light and dark, turn to page 98. You can also use a wearable light therapy device called the Re-Timer (re-timer.com), which helps your body naturally adjust to your preferred sleep time by harnessing the power of light.

When you stay online late at night, your mind continues to whir when you eventually switch off the lights.

SYNC YOURSELF **WITH THE SUN**

WHAT HAPPENS WHEN YOU TAKE A RHYTHMIC HUMAN OUT OF THEIR NATURAL WILDERNESS ENVIRONMENT AND PLOP THEM RIGHT IN THE MIDDLE OF *TODAY*—AN ELECTRICITY-FILLED LANDSCAPE, ABUZZ AND ABLAZE WITH LIT SCREENS AND STREAMING INFORMATION? THEIR BRAINS GET ALL THE WRONG SIGNALS AND

RESTORATIVE SLEEP CAN GO OUT THE WINDOW! Adjusting your exposure to light and dark is the most powerful way to impose some old-fashioned order and find harmonious sleep patterns again, without returning to the bush (though that helps—see page 106). Exposing yourself to light and dark at the proper times helps regulate your sleep cycle, and how well you will sleep tonight will be partly decided by what you do this morning. Practice these basic daylight protocols to get your fill of light, at the right time.

EXPOSE YOURSELF TO LIGHT RIGHT AWAY. If your sleep patterns are in disarray, go for a brief walk in daylight as soon as you wake (another good reason to have a dog, page 215). Your internal clock is especially sensitive to the energizing effects of light in the first two hours after waking.

GET OUTSIDE SEVERAL TIMES THROUGHOUT THE DAY (you need to get your movement in—see page 120—so it's a win-win!). Small exposures to natural light will help maximize alertness while increasing vitamin D absorption. Leave your sunglasses off, so light directly hits your eyes. Even cloudy days expose you to greater intensity of light than the average artificially lit office. And lose the shoes (page 161)! Barefoot contact with nature, aka "earthing," restores balanced cortisol and can help you find your sleep rhythm.

IF OUTDOOR TIME IS LIMITED, CONSIDER SITTING FOR 30 TO 90 MINUTES A DAY IN FRONT OF FULL-SPECTRUM LIGHTS, often used to treat seasonal affective disorder (SAD) and other circadian-related mood and sleep disorders. Put one on your desk and let it bathe you in light as you work. (Brookstone makes a good one.)

FIND A SMALL WINDOW OF TIME TO UNWIND and shed stress. Try a short meditation (page 194) or the rituals suggested in How to Get Ready for Bed (page 110).

ANTICIPATE YOUR EVENING TO COME. What do you have to get done before lights out? What nonnegotiable tasks (or nonnegotiable entertainment) might have you sitting in front of your computer after dinner? How else could you plan your evening so that your after-dark hours are, well, a little darker (page 102)? Looking ahead can help you succeed in starting new habits.

Adjusting your exposure to light and dark is the most powerful way to find harmonious sleep patterns.

RESTORE YOUR ANCESTRAL
CONNECTION TO DARK

AH, DARKNESS. HOW FAR WE'VE COME FROM OUR ANCESTRAL NORM, WHEN THE HOURS AFTER SUNSET WOULD HAVE ONLY BEEN LIT (AFTER THE ADVENT OF FIRE, THAT IS) BY THE GLOWING RED LIGHT OF BURNING LOGS, THE STARS, AND THE MOON. SINCE THERE WAS NOTHING MUCH TO DO IN THE DARK SAVE HUNKER DOWN

OUT OF SIGHT OF PREDATORS, SLEEP WOULD OCCUR soon after night fell. There would be no light again until sunrise. Our evolutionary DNA—the cellular information that determines how we function—knows true dark well.

But our modern minds and lifestyles don't! Today, once night falls and any kids are (hopefully) in bed, the busyness begins. We get busy in the kitchen, busy catching up on work or catching up with our lives, and it all happens under a wash of omnipresent, artificial light. And it's not just indoors: Our previously dark surroundings are now lit up, and our once mysterious starry skies are aglow with cityscape glare. Experts say there's been a tenfold increase in the amount of artificial light used per capita in the last fifty years, and that nights are bright in a way that, quite frankly, confounds our biology (some have gone so far as to label outdoor light pollution a human health risk). Consequently, our internal clocks run three to five hours later than in caveperson days, when we might have been asleep at 7:00 p.m. Yet we typically can't sleep in to compensate for the loss—that giant lag would make anyone fatigued.

Excessive exposure to artificial light at night, particularly blue light, has been linked to increased risks for obesity, depression, sleep disorders, diabetes, and breast cancer. Biologists know that artificial light at night has terrible effects on nocturnal animals and migrating animals, birds, and insects. Why wouldn't it be similarly disruptive for us?

Tempering your exposure to light at night, and ensuring a state of "true dark" when you sleep, is a crucial step in restoring rhythms and ensuring sleep wellness. Though only fringe health-seekers take it seriously right now—it's

this crowd that's sparked the trend for wearing "blue-blocker" glasses at night—I predict that following healthy night-lighting behavior will someday be considered as important as eating your vegetables. The more you can approximate preindustrial light conditions, the better your sleep will be, and it *is* possible to do this while still enjoying your home and life. Here's how to harness the power of dark to improve your sleep.

1. **CREATE AN ELECTRONIC SUNDOWN.** The single most important light exposure correction is to power down devices a couple hours before bedtime. This shields your eyes from blue light and lets your mind wind down. Install an orange-light app such as f.lux on your computer, use an app such as Night Filter for Android devices, or switch to Night Shift on your iPhone or iPad. (Other "evening" options are available for e-readers.) You can also purchase physical shields for computers and phones that protect your eyes from the damaging and straining effects of LED lights, made by a company called Reticare. And turn down the brightness of your screen: If you do end up plugged in and switched on at night, your device will at least cast a less-disrupting sunset-mimicking light.

2. **MAKE YOUR BEDROOM GLOW.** If you wind down in your bedroom and read before sleep, replace the light bulbs by your bedside with amber-toned bulbs. You can get an amber-toned LED that will last for thousands of hours, or a HealthE Sleepy Baby bulb designed to keep babies dozing during nighttime diaper changes! Another option: a pink Himalayan salt lamp, which emits a gentle glow while, proponents say, helping to purify air of mold and bacteria,

and mildly counteracting the "positive ion" impact of electronics. (Test it for yourself—many people report feeling better with these lamps in their homes.)

3. **DIM THE LIGHTS ELSEWHERE.** The truth of the matter is that any blue-wave light will stimulate your circadian rhythm the wrong way. Which means if you're in the kitchen until 11:00 p.m., working under LED spotlights, it's going to be harder to wind down. Dimming the lights in your home will help, but your best bet is to complete "brightly lit" activities earlier in the evening, then spend your last two hours before bed in a softly lit sanctuary. Use low incandescent lights, amber lamps, salt lamps, or glow lights; you can also use candles to emit a campfire glow, which has a profoundly soothing effect! There is even "smart lighting" that connects bulbs to smart home systems to create an amber wash of light at night.

4. **TO ENSURE APPROPRIATELY TIMED MELATONIN RELEASE, YOU CAN WEAR "BLUE-BLOCKER" GLASSES,** which have orange lenses (the kind made for industrial protection) for the pre-bed hours! You won't win any style prizes, but at $10 a pop, they're worth a try if sleepy feelings elude you. The caveat: You must keep them on until all bright or white lights are out, even while brushing your teeth.

5. **SURVEY YOUR BEDROOM FOR UNWELCOME LIGHT.** Since the receptors in your eyes are photosensitive when you're asleep, illumination from the street outside your windows, and glowing lights on alarm clocks, gadgets, and air-conditioners, all can disrupt your sleep rhythm. Do a light detox: Make your bedroom a light-proof sanctuary by fixing light seepage through your blinds or curtains (see page 109); remove electronics (turn your alarm clock around or, better yet, replace it with analog); and cover any remaining blips of electronic light with duct tape.

6. **USE A VERY LOW-WATTAGE NIGHT LIGHT IN YOUR BATHROOM** if you need to get up in the night. Don't turn on the overhead lights—even brief exposure will disrupt melatonin and make returning to sleep harder.

WHAT'S THE ISSUE WITH MY LIGHT BULB?

In a nutshell, the issue is that white, artificial light is high in shorter-wavelength blue light, just like natural daylight. When the sensors in the eye see blue light, they signal the SCN (page 98) that it's daytime—time to wake up! Some of the "bluest" artificial lights are the LED lights used in light bulbs and our computer and gadget screens—even compact fluorescent lights (CFLs) have a blue wash to them. Conversely, the amber glow of candles and fires is longer-wavelength red light. It mimics the light of sunset and, as a result, cues your master clock to trigger sleep.

7. **DON'T GLANCE AT YOUR CELL PHONE TO FIND OUT THE TIME IN THE DARKNESS.** That hit of brightness will be like a shot of espresso to your brain, even if it's just for a few seconds while setting your alarm. Leave the cell phone outside the room. (If you want to use your phone for music, white noise, or a sleep app, see page 114.)

8. **MINIMIZE ANY SURROUNDING LIGHT POLLUTION YOU CAN.** Use outdoor lighting only where necessary—add motion detectors or timers, or change the angle of lights. Need help cleaning up excess light from your surroundings? Check out darksky.org for resources on how to help minimize light pollution in your neighborhood as well as contribute to citizen science on the issue.

CLOSE YOUR EYES, CLEAN YOUR BRAIN

Sleep is not a luxury; it is an absolutely essential act of daily maintenance, and it is your ally in keeping your brain sharp and youthful.

NEXT TIME YOU'RE ABOUT TO CHEAT YOURSELF OF sleep, consider this: Sleep may be pivotal to avoiding early mental decline. When you sleep, your brain protects itself from toxic proteins. Its glymphatic system flushes cerebrospinal fluid through the brain to remove proteins that accumulate between the cells as a byproduct of neurological processes during the day (it is the equivalent of the lymphatic system in the body). This "overnight cleanup" keeps the brain clear and healthy, but it only occurs when you're asleep—it's as if you have a brain-cleaning crew who only works the night shift. If, by depriving yourself of solid sleep, you don't let them work, it's like having a party one night and neglecting to clean the mess the next day, and then having another party. These waste products begin to accumulate, and the house starts deteriorating. Science is now linking this toxic buildup with loss of neurological function. You might feel a state of brain fog or have poor memory, or find your cognitive performance declines (if you've become absentminded after chronic sleep disruption, this may be why). Over time, this "trash buildup" of proteins in the brain can even contribute to dementia and Alzheimer's.

Given how active our brains are today, thinking, solving, and creating on a continuous loop, having this disposal system in tip-top shape feels more important than ever. Sleep (as well as its deeply restful counterpart, meditation) is not a luxury; it is an absolutely essential act of daily maintenance, and it is your ally in keeping your brain sharp and youthful. Don't skimp on it!

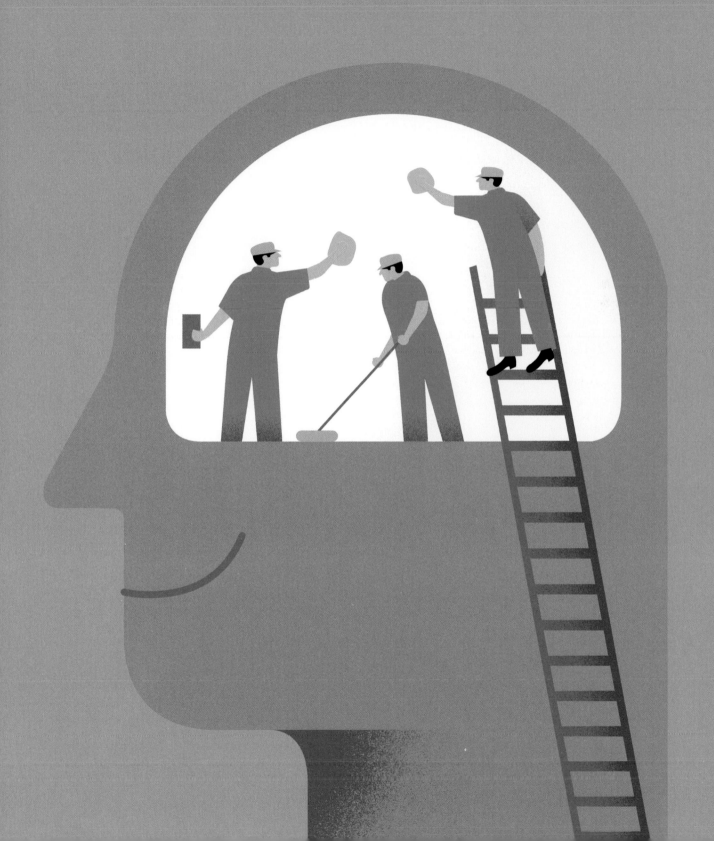

STAR **RX**

HUMANS HAVE A PHYSIOLOGICAL NEED TO BE IMMERSED IN OUTDOOR DARKNESS. THIS IS BOTH A BIOLOGI-CAL AND, I BELIEVE, SPIRITUAL NEED. A RECENT STUDY TOOK A GROUP OF CAMPERS INTO THE COLORADO ROCKIES FOR A WEEK, WHERE THEY HAD NO ACCESS TO LIGHT AT NIGHT EXCEPT FOR THEIR EVENING CAMPFIRE.

VERY QUICKLY, THEY BEGAN FALLING ASLEEP EARLIER and sleeping for longer periods; their bodies had adjusted to the natural rhythms of light and dark. It took no extra effort on their part, and the regulated rhythms lasted when they returned home. No-frills camping, it seems, is a potent medicine for improving dysregulated sleep patterns!

But it's more than that. Experiencing the night deeply gives you something intangible yet meaningful. A sense of wonder. A sense of perspective. As the Connect ring shows, this is as vital to being well as any nutrient or exercise.

If you live in a town or city, immersing yourself in the night may feel like a risky endeavor, or a fruitless one since so much artificial light filters upward, drowning stars. But it's a powerful prescription to keep in your pocket, whether you get a chance to truly Go Wild (page 216) and find the blackest sky around, or you join a group night experience closer to home—a full-moon hike in a local park, an outdoor astronomy class hosted by a local science center, or even an outdoor concert or festival where you can lose yourself in darkness, surrounded by your tribe (page 234). We weren't designed to be as cut off from the night sky in the ways we are today. Try this simple practice once or twice, and see how it affects your awareness of how natural light and natural dark affect your body and mind.

Find astronomy clubs near you at lovethenightsky.com.

Whether you know it or not, sleep is anything but unproductive — your brain and body are actually very active when you're down for the count.

DE-DIGITIZE YOUR NIGHT

THE EVIDENCE IS IRREFUTABLE. IF YOU WANT TO SLEEP BETTER, TAKE BACK CONTROL OF AFTER-DARK TECH HABITS. GETTING HOOKED IN TO DIGITAL MEDIA AND INFORMATION—FROM INNOCENTLY WATCHING YOUR FAVORITE SHOWS (ON A BIG SCREEN OR SMALL) TO SCROLLING THROUGH SOCIAL MEDIA—SQUELCHES SLEEP

TRIGGERS, NOT JUST BECAUSE OF LIGHT DISRUPTION, but also because it promotes alertness and mental revving. Sure, these activities make you feel you are sinking into some hard-earned "me time" and unwinding, and today's mediascape, which allows binge-watching at any time, doesn't make it easy to unplug. But think of it this way: These innocent-seeming habits reverse your body's natural downturn toward sleep.

Even if you change your screens to orange (page 102), you're not in the clear. Start noticing how watching a show when you begin to feel sleepy can arrest the downward dive your body has started. Suddenly, you're not so tired. Or notice that when you stay online late at night, your mind continues to whir when you eventually switch off the lights.

For years, eastern healers have advised not to even read books before bed! The idea is that any stimulating mental activity hinders sleep. In today's world, we've sprinted far past books, and the effects are catching up with us.

 Our Be Well integrative psychiatrist, **Ellen Vora, MD,** counsels extensively on sleep and technology issues and has this to say:

Falling down the electronic rabbit hole at night is like binging on pizza: The temptation gets put before you, it sucks you in, triggering you to consume it mindlessly, and then you feel icky the next day. Today's apps are designed to get you scrolling infinitely—your brain expects to arrive at an ending,

but there isn't one, and that's what gets you into trouble. Bring consciousness to your choices of how you spend your time at night. If you're going to stare at a screen, know that it may impact your sleep, so enter that agreement mindfully. Sometimes it's necessary, but for those times when it's not, don't just be on autopilot and default to scanning Instagram. Four ways to develop this self-awareness are:

1. SET AN ALARM THAT MEANS TECHNOLOGY TIME IS OVER and it's time to start unwinding—and don't press snooze.

2. MAKE SOMEONE YOU LIVE WITH—PARTNER OR ROOMMATE—AN ACCOUNTABILITY PARTNER. If you see each other going down the rabbit hole, gently note what you observe. You'll snap at each other at first, but it will help.

3. REMEMBER THAT SLEEP IS ESSENTIAL FOR PRODUCTIVITY. Burning the midnight oil won't help the quality of your work as much as falling asleep by 10:30 p.m. will.

4. JUST LIKE WITH FOOD, PAY HEED TO HOW YOU FEEL THE MORNING AFTER a late-night tech session steals your sleep and disrupts its quality. Notice if your brain or body feels the impact, or how your morning goes. Let awareness fuel your commitment to do things differently the next night.

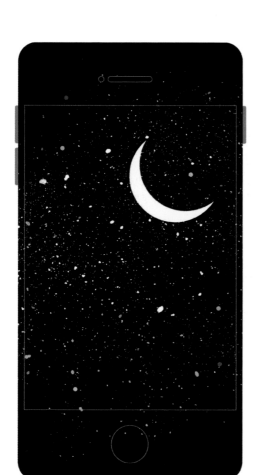

SECRETS OF SUCCESSFUL SLEEPERS

SUCCESSFUL SLEEPERS . . .

. . . GO TO BED WHEN THEY'RE TIRED. Babies get over-tired and impossible to soothe, and adults do, too. Push through your natural sleepy signals to stay up late and you'll toss and turn that night.

. . . DON'T EAT THEIR EVENING MEALS TOO LATE. To stay in sync with your sleep-inducing rhythms, eat dinner at least two to three hours before bedtime (see page 79) and avoid sugar at night. When an after-dinner craving or hunger pang strikes, have a spoonful of quality almond butter to help stabilize your blood sugar. Dips in blood sugar can also be a cause of middle-of-the-night wake-fulness. If so, repeat the spoonful.

. . . AVOID ALCOHOL CLOSE TO BEDTIME. Booze might make you drowsy (unless it's tequila, which does the opposite), but it's a poor crutch, because it can actually delay the onset of REM sleep, which means the restorative quality of sleep suffers. Limit alcohol to one drink, and have it at least three hours before bedtime so your body can process the alcohol. If you notice that even a little alcohol with dinner disrupts your sleep, pour a bit of tart cherry juice in your wineglass instead of wine. It contains a small amount of melatonin.

. . . LEAVE TECHNOLOGY (AND TV) OUT OF THE BED-ROOM. It's an oldie but a goodie: Keep your bedroom reserved for sleep and sex.

. . . HAVE THE WI-FI ROUTER ON A TIMER. This limits the temptation to go online before bed and protects you from disruptive electromagnetic frequency, which new research shows is more pernicious when you sleep. See page 165 for more on this.

. . . SLEEP IN A VERY DARK ROOM. Assess whether hormone-disrupting light from outside is leaking in through your window treatments. Blackout curtains or shades are a great investment—and surprisingly affordable through services like Home Depot's—though you can find some innovative (albeit un-chic) ways to hack this online. The cheap fix, if you can't control your room environment: a good eye mask that stays on while you sleep.

. . . STAY COMFORTABLY COOL AT NIGHT. It has been proven that you sleep better in a room that is around 60 to 67 degrees Fahrenheit. When you sleep, your body temperature naturally drops. A cooler room (and a hot bath, page 110) can help you get there. It's better to crack the window and snuggle under a thicker cover than to turn up the heat; in summer, keep your room on the cooler side. If your extremities get chilly, wear socks in bed or place a hot water bottle at your feet. It will warm your feet without raising your core temperature.

. . . WORK IT OUT WITH THEIR PARTNER. Ensure that one person isn't waving around an iPad while the other is trying to snooze. Agreeing to limit technology in the bedroom can be a nonpersonal way to engender compromise. If your partner wakes you by moving, consider investing in a good mattress with minimal "transference" of movement. If snoring is the issue, ear plugs and a white noise machine can help, as well as gently supporting the snorer to look at possible causes such as food sensitivities, allergies, alcohol consumption, and weight gain.

. . . USE AN ALTERNATIVE ALARM CLOCK. Once your glowing cell phone (and its alarm feature) is banished and your ultrabright digital alarm clock is unplugged, you need another option. Cheap battery-operated travel alarms are an easy alternative. But so are "light" alarms that gradually illuminate, mimicking the dawn, or chime alarms that increase in volume from subtle to loud, such as the one made by Now & Zen. Both are stress-free ways to get woken.

. . . DON'T GO TO SLEEP ANGRY. Disallow fearful, angry, or resentful thinking after lights-out. These thoughts literally "switch on" the stress response and can trigger cortisol release (the hormone of alertness and hyper-vigilance). A positive affirmation or a gratitude practice can create an inhospitable environment for those sneaky thoughts.

>>

Some reasons to make sleep a priority: it's when your body repairs, restores, maintains, and detoxifies itself. How you sleep is as important as how you live during waking hours.

<<

HOW TO GET
READY FOR BED

YOU CAN'T GO AT FULL SPEED ALL DAY AND THEN SUDDENLY STOP, DROP, AND SLEEP. CREATE A BUFFER ZONE BETWEEN ACTION AND REST—BETWEEN DAYTIME'S YANG ENERGY OF DOING AND ACHIEVING, AND NIGHTTIME'S YIN STATE OF INWARD STILLNESS—WITH THESE RELIABLE RITUALS FOR TRANSITIONING

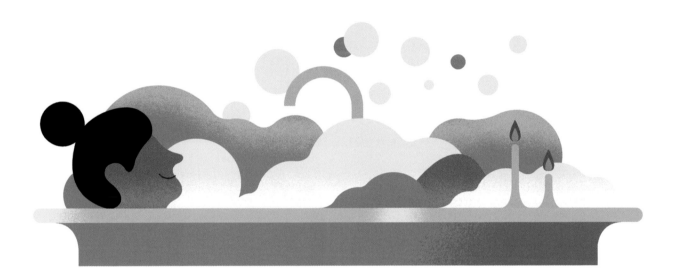

TO TRANQUILITY. CHILDREN SLEEP BETTER WHEN they have a consistent pre-bed routine. Adults aren't all that different.

TAKE A BATH. A hot shower or bath before bed makes your core temperature drop as your blood circulates to your periphery. This helps trigger sleep because a cooling body temperature is a natural part of your sleep rhythm. Doctor up your bath with Epsom salts, which infuse rest-inducing and muscle-relaxing magnesium into your tissues, helping to mitigate stress and inflammation. Lavender

oil added to the bath, a tried-and-tested classic, also induces relaxation.

MAKE A HEALTHY NIGHTCAP. Herbal teas and tonics have been used for eons to gently help the nervous system shift from revved to relaxed. Chamomile is the classic go-to, but there's a profusion of nighttime blends available, and some popular powdered mixes that use Chinese herbs. Not everyone responds the same way to each of these; personal exploration is the only way to find what works for you. If you are curious about trying herbs in a more targeted way for sleep, visit a local herb store (or online retailer like mountainroseherbs.com). Consider using skullcap, which relaxes and restores the nervous system, if your sleep ghoul is anxiety; California poppy if the problem is that your mind is running; or valerian, passionflower, or magnolia if you tend to wake up and can't fall back asleep. (As with all herbs, get professional guidance if you are pregnant or on medication.) For extra help, you might also consider taking magnesium or some of the more targeted sleep supplements outlined on page 112.

USE MUSIC. Though it's fairly obvious if you've ever sung a lullaby to a baby, studies show that the right kind of pre-bed music can significantly improve sleep quality when used consistently—even for those with chronic sleep disorders. We don't yet fully know the exact mechanisms that music triggers that help induce sleep, but we know it can boost the brain's pleasure centers while lowering physiological arousal, and it can release endogenous opioids (your natural pain killers) and oxytocin (the hormone of bonding). Both physical and emotional pain—which could be the root of sleep disorder for some—appear to be alleviated.

Though soothing, slower-paced classical and reggae music are two ways to go, there's now a treasure chest of music that is crafted to help you drop more easily into a slow-brainwave state. In particular, music using binaural beats help the electrical activity in the brain slow down by merging two different frequencies. This allows your brain to experience a much lower frequency of sound than it can normally hear. Hemi-Sync (hemi-sync.com) is a system that helps brainwaves slow down for sleep, and the vanguard "music as medicine" platform Sync Project (syncproject.co) offers a whole category of sound and music devoted to slumber.

DO RESTORATIVE YOGA. Pick one or two postures from page 206 and let them be the last thing you do before climbing into bed. They work by switching on the rest and relax functions of the nervous system. Dim lights and calming music can enhance the experience. For a guided experience, visit supersleepyoga.com, an online course designed to help trigger sleep (and help you get back to sleep if you wake up in the night).

PRACTICE LETTING GO. As you lie in bed with the lights out, try spending three to ten minutes doing a simple practice that combines body awareness with breathing. You can begin by using the 4-7-8 breath (page 185) to relax, and then, moving upward from toes to head, including the belly, chest, heart, and arms, inwardly thank each body part for their efforts today, telling them they can rest. Feel each body part sink into the bed as you let go. For guidance, look up body scan meditations on YouTube. After you hear them a few times, you will able to do them easily on your own.

Disallow fearful, angry, or resentful thinking after lights-out. These thoughts literally "switch on" the stress response.

BEAT THE NO-SLEEP BLUES

PRACTICING GOOD SLEEP HYGIENE AND BEING CONSCIOUS OF EVENING HABITS DOES NOT ALWAYS GUARANTEE PERFECT SLEEP. IF YOU HAVE INSOMNIA—OCCASIONALLY OR FREQUENTLY—YOU MIGHT BE PAINFULLY AWARE OF THIS FACT, AND WITH THE LEVEL OF STRESS AND ANXIETY PERVADING OUR LIVES,

LACK OF SLEEP IS ON THE RISE. TODAY, MEDICATIONS for sleep are a hugely growing business (predicted to hit $80 billion globally by 2020), but while pharmaceutical drugs may help initially, they increase your risk for dementia, are addictive, and can cause bizarre behaviors.

Though there's rarely a quick fix for this incredibly debilitating experience, addressing the following areas can help to lessen insomnia's grip.

NORMALIZE WAKING UP. If you experience mild wakefulness occasionally and can get back to sleep without struggle, you don't need to worry. Research shows that throughout evolutionary history, it's been normal to wake up in the night. The problem can start if you stress about it and then can't quiet your mind.

CUT BACK ON CAFFEINE. Individual sensitivity to caffeine varies widely, but few people realize that this drug can stay in your system for more than seven hours after you consume it. It's crucial to curb caffeine if you struggle with sleep: Dial back the amount you consume, and never drink it after noon. If you need a coffee fix in the afternoon, try a caffeine-free alternative like herbal coffee made with dandelion and chicory root.

DON'T TAKE SUPPLEMENTS AFTER 5:00 P.M. While some people metabolize vitamins and other supplements fine at night, others get wakeful. With the exception of calming magnesium or other sleep blends, take your supplements by lunchtime unless you know they won't affect you.

MOVE AND EXERCISE DAILY. People who exercise at least 150 minutes a week report twice the likelihood of satisfying sleep than nonexercisers. And consider strength-training programs: For your muscles to repair themselves after working out, they demand growth hormone that is secreted in deep sleep, which is why bodybuilders often report profound slumber. If you exercise in the evening, finish by 7:00 or 8:00 p.m. in order to allow time for winding down.

KEEP DAYTIME NAPS SHORT. If you are tired enough to nap during the day, do it before 4:00 p.m. and keep it limited to twenty to thirty minutes so you don't enter a deep sleep cycle, which can disrupt nighttime sleep.

SUPPLEMENT FOR SLEEP. The entry-level supplements to help sleep are either magnesium citrate powder or magnesium glycinate or threonate (start with 300mg and increase to 400 or 500mg if needed) and glycine (start with 3g and increase if needed). You can try them individually or mixed together in water. (The magnesium citrate will have a loosening/encouraging effect on the bowels.) If these aren't effective, try L-theanine and GABA. Individuals react differently to each, so some trial and error may be required. Start with at least 200 to 400mg L-theanine or 300 to 600mg GABA and see which one works for you. A combination of the two can also work well.

IF YOU WAKE, DON'T LIE IN BED TOSSING AND TURNING. With the lights still out, put on calming music (page 191) or an audio book, or try the body scan meditation technique (page 111).

GET CHECKED FOR SLEEP APNEA. If you constantly wake up exhausted, ask your doctor about sleep apnea. This fairly common condition interferes with your ability to breathe while you sleep, preventing you from getting deep sleep. It is potentially dangerous but easily treated at home with machines that are now smaller and more accessible than before.

REVIEW YOUR MEDICATIONS. Antihistamines, diuretics, antipsychotics, antidepressants, decongestants, asthma medications, and some blood pressure medicines can cause sleeplessness and disturb REM sleep. Ask your doctor or pharmacist if what you're taking might be interfering with your sleep.

TRY A FLOAT TANK. These increasingly popular remedies for stress and pain can help reduce cortisol levels and inflammation, often helping to restore easier sleep. For about an hour during the day, you simply lie in a silent pod filled with water loaded with 1,000 pounds of Epsom salts and let the womblike environment work its calming magic. There are dedicated float tank centers popping up nationwide, and you can also find them at some spas.

CONSIDER CHRONOTHERAPY. If you cannot fall asleep until after 2:00 a.m. no matter how many changes you make, look into chronotherapy, a therapeutic regimen that uses light to help reset your circadian rhythms. It has also been shown to help with the depression that is so often related to sleep disorders.

While pharmaceutical sleep aids may help initially, they increase your risk for dementia, are addictive, and can cause bizarre behaviors.

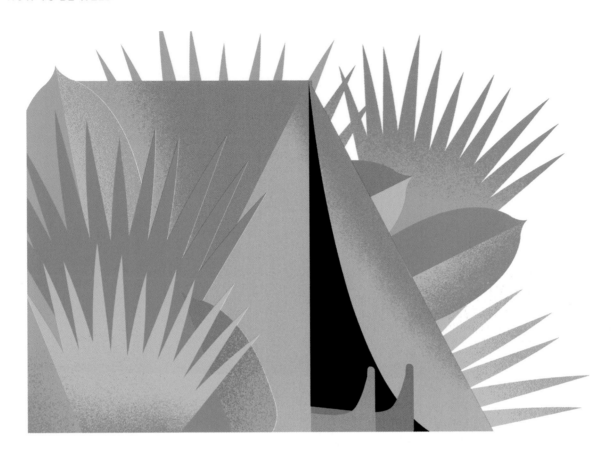

EXPLORE THE NEW FRONTIERS
(THEN GO TO SLEEP!)

SLEEP TECHNOLOGY IS A BOOMING INDUSTRY. THERE ARE BETTER BEDS, BETTER SHEETS, AND NOW A TIDAL WAVE OF APPS, PROGRAMS, AND DEVICES THAT PROMISE SWEET SLUMBER. TRACKERS CAN BE USEFUL ALLIES IN GETTING SOME INFORMATION ABOUT SLEEP PATTERNS, THOUGH THE JURY'S STILL OUT REGARDING THE

ACCURACY OF THEIR DATA. (A SLEEP LAB IS THE REAL way to dive deeply into sleep dysfunction.) And do you want devices that may emit EMFs (electromagnetic fields) next to your head all night? If you use a sleep app to drift off, remember to set your phone to airplane mode and ideally connect it to a speaker away from your immediate reach so you're not tempted to grab your phone if you wake up in the night.

Think of all of these as short-term strategies for gathering information or instilling new habits. No gadget is going to override accumulated stress you have not shed or be more effective than tiring out your muscles with a workout. The goal is to be able to get good z's without accessories and interventions. At the end of the day, we evolved to lie down on bare ground, in the dark, without much on our mind, and sleep.

\>\>

When your sleep goes awry, it's a clue that something about your lifestyle is asking to be adjusted, or that something else in your body needs attention.

\<\<

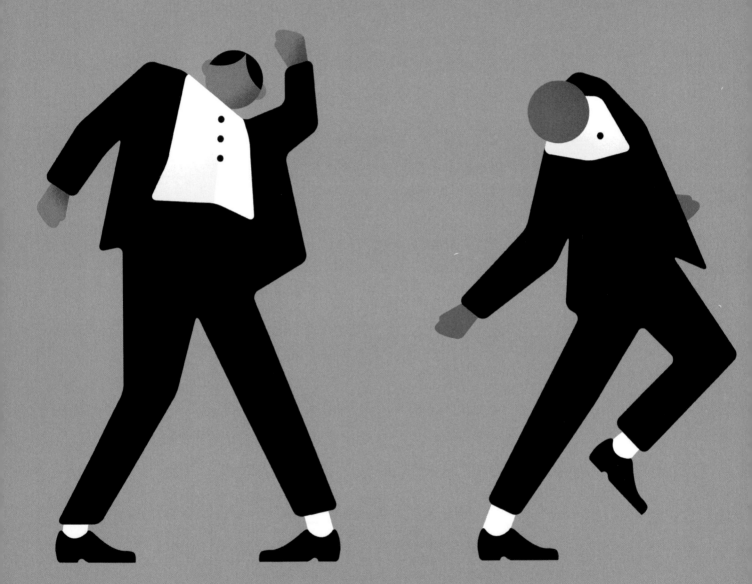

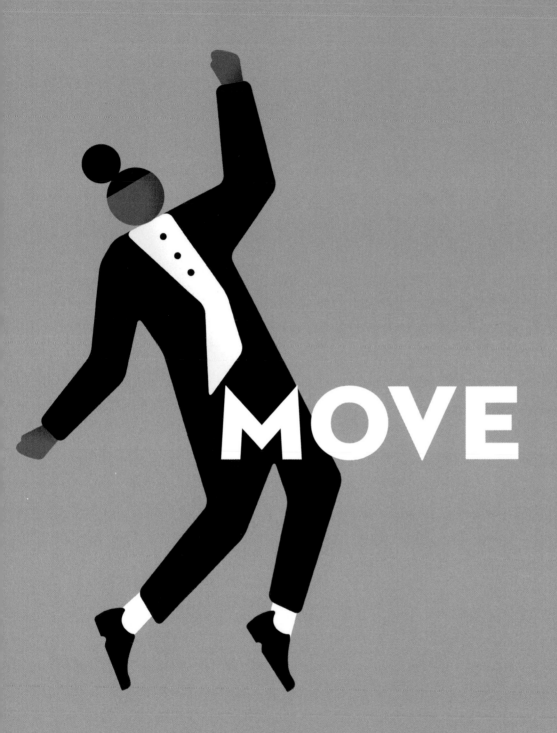

MOVE

THIS RING OF THE MANDALA IS NOT CALLED "WORK Out." It's *Move*. Before there were gyms, treadmills, and sneakers, there was simple human movement. For most of human history, your forebears did a lot of it. All day, most days, in fact (six miles of walking for food and water per day, it is said).

The irony of our highly "mobile" culture is that while we can take our work with us and stay connected wherever we go, actual movement has been downgraded. We sit. And we sit. If we're lucky, we get some isolated bursts of exercise—though for many, even that's become a bit of an artifact.

The Move ring is not about urgently pursuing fitness or burning calories per se (when it comes to weight management, you can't out-exercise a poor diet). It's about integrating movement back into your day so you can use (and enjoy) your body the way nature intended it: as a vehicle capable of carrying you comfortably through the life you want to live. A practice of dedicated body training fits into this, but it's built on slow gains, steady progress, and a foundation of smart eating and sound sleep.

Moving improves *everything:* your metabolism and your microbiome, your sleep and all your body rhythms, your immunity, your stress response, and the overall balance in your life. It even decreases inflammation. You don't have to be a rock-star cyclist or sculpt a body of steel. Just ask yourself, upon waking, "How can I move more today?"

FIND THE MOVEMENT
THAT MOVES YOU

WHAT IF YOU REFRAMED THE IDEA OF WORKING OUT FROM BEING A CHORE TO A PRACTICE: A RELATIONSHIP THAT SUSTAINS YOU, NOURISHES YOU, AND SOMETIMES JUST HOLDS YOU IN A PLACE OF RELIEF OR REST? BE WELL COLLABORATOR SADIE LINCOLN IS THE FOUNDER AND CEO OF THE BARRE3 WORKOUT, WHICH DEVELOPS

HOW TO BE WELL EXPERT BALANCED, STRONG BODIES, AND AN ADVOcate of bringing a movement practice into your life. I'm a big fan of Sadie's mindful and functional methodology, which fuses ballet barre, Pilates, and yoga. It's a different philosophy toward exercise, and it may look a little different than forcing yourself to go to the gym. She shares how a small shift in attitude can lead to sticking to something for the long term and enjoying it, too:

Having a consistent *practice* of something you love to do lets you reclaim movement as a part of your integrated way of being, versus it being something that you need to "achieve." It's a completely different mindset from trying to meet some kind of perfected fitness ideal, which is where we've been for decades. That often leads you to strive to a goal that is not authentic to who you are—one that's either shaped by an impossible industry standard, or comes from your own ideal of yourself from a previous, athletic time in your life!

The key to developing a long-lasting movement practice is that it be something that grows your own body awareness, and an ability to know where you are in that moment; it will change from day to day, depending on how *you* are feeling, and what you know you need. A challenging experience one day; breathing and mobility the next. The type of practice could be anything—from a barre3 class or yoga practice to Olympic lifting   but the teacher should teach a methodology where you learn to adapt movements according to your strengths and weaknesses so you link present-moment awareness with your movement. Look around the room: Is everyone doing slightly different versions of the pose or exercise? That's

a clue that you're on the right track. Because that's where the magic happens; you start to really know "What do I need today?" Our bodies are ever in constant change. So is the world we live in. So why would our movement practice stay the same? This approach—a more mindful approach—may not be as high-octane as you expect at first. But stick with it! We've all been conditioned to be sensation junkies—"no pain, no gain." Replace that old thinking with "work smarter, not harder." That's how you learn to be your own best teacher.

Start by finding something you connect to and have fun with—try things out online to see if they pique your interest. Then get to a class if you possibly can, because the community and culture of group movement is just as important as the practice itself. Seek a teacher who lives to see you, rather than performs for you. Do they remember your name and look you in the eye? Do they give a hands-on adjustment and ask you questions? Whether it be a barre studio, a dojo, a yoga shala, a climbing gym, or something else, this group environment gives you a very powerful tool for modern life: a tool for fighting loneliness. There's nothing like exploring the experience of movement, together.

JUST MOVE
(AS MUCH AS YOU CAN)

WORKOUTS ARE ENRICHING, EMPOWERING, AND IF YOU WANT TO ACHIEVE PEAK PHYSICAL POTENTIAL, PROBABLY A REQUISITE. BUT THEY'RE NOT THE BE-ALL, END-ALL. THOUGH SIXTY MINUTES OF AN EXERCISE CLASS OR GYM SESSION IS A POSITIVE INPUT, HOURS OF IMMOBILITY BEFORE AND AFTER NOT ONLY CAN EAT

UP THE GAINS—LEAVING YOU FRUSTRATED WITH your lack of progress or your ratio of fat to muscle—they might cause you to reinforce the small pains and physical glitches of your chair-bound body because the tiny micro-tears that come from lifting weights can heal in that shape. Don't ditch a workout that you enjoy, but if you're sweating about making it to the gym at the crack of dawn, it might be better to try to get more movement throughout the day.

YOU ARE DESIGNED TO MOVE

Your physical mechanics, brilliantly evolved over many millennia, are designed for many activities: to walk frequently and for some distance; to change physical planes (by standing up and then sitting back down, and by pivoting, turning, or lunging in multiple directions); and to pull, push, and hoist things (even if just the weight of your body) regularly. This allows your joints to stay lubricated and injury-free and your tendons to remain robust (and able to handle loads of weight or unexpected movements), and it ensures that all the components of your skeletal and muscular systems move fluidly, without soreness and restriction. You are also protected: Movement causes muscle tissue to produce proteins called myokines that have important disease-preventive and anti-inflammation functions.

What happens when this brilliantly designed machine stops moving? A lifestyle change of such epic proportions that it delivers a host of unwanted side effects. Apart from the obvious discomfort and stiffness of restricted mobility, a sedentary lifestyle is associated with higher cancer risk, depression, lower cognitive ability, pre-diabetic blood sugar levels (even at a healthy weight), diminished sex life and reproductive health, sleep disruption and insomnia, and an epidemic of disc degeneration and resulting back pain. The shift to a sedentary culture has taken an enormous toll.

We live in boxes, travel in boxes, eat out of boxes, and work in boxes—now it's time to urgently break out of the box! That's easier said than done when limiting factors

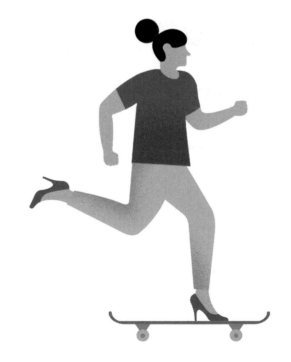

(such as a job, commute, or dependents) determine your schedule. But it's possible to get crafty even within those limitations. Find the small windows of time for weaving physical activity throughout your waking hours. Whether you make it to an actual workout, run, or bike ride—and chances are high that many days you will not—you will have taken solid steps to promote and protect your health. Use all the tips in this ring to help you, and integrate the following approaches into your everyday:

MAKE MOVEMENT A HEALTHY BYPRODUCT OF MEETING OTHER NEEDS. If you have kids, take them out to roam and explore, or if they're very small, wear them and get out for a walk. If you're doing errands, ditch the car a few blocks before your destination and walk the final distance. If you drive to work, is there an alternative route that would get you to walk or bike, at least part of the way?

SHIFT THE WAY YOU WORK. Do phone calls have to take place while seated? A headset and pad of paper could free you up to make calls on the move. And who said that meetings must take place in the boardroom? Creativity and collaboration can flow better when the body is in motion—cross-body movements like walking actually stimulate exchange of information between the hemispheres of the brain.

REFRESH YOUR SOCIAL LIFE. Commit to walking or playing sports with friends instead of catching up over coffee or dinner. If it's after dark, try something like yoga, dance, or mixed martial arts.

MAKE A GAME OF YOUR COMMUTE. If you work on a high floor in an office building, try this drill: Every day for a week, get off the elevator before your floor, dropping a floor each day, *every single time you go in and out*. Monday: Get off one floor early. Tuesday: two floors early. Wednesday: three floors. And so on.

WALK FIVE BLOCKS BEFORE LUNCH. Take a stroll before eating, and if you're getting takeout, don't order in—pick it up! Not only does this add steps to your day, it improves insulin sensitivity slightly, decompresses your digestive system, and destresses your nervous system in prepara-

tion for your meal, and makes you more wakeful so you are less likely to crave pick-me-up sugars.

EMBRACE MICRO SESSIONS. Do any kind of movement for ten minutes at least once or twice a day. Ten minutes can change your state completely—it's just three songs on a pop playlist. (If you think you don't have ten minutes, sacrifice checking your social media and grab that time back!)

A sedentary lifestyle is associated with higher cancer risk, depression, lower cognitive ability, prediabetic blood sugar levels, diminshed sex life, and sleep disruption.

GET STRONG!

STRENGTH CONFERS RESILIENCE, LONGEVITY, AND PROTECTION AGAINST DISEASE. BUT UNLESS YOU HAVE SOME KIND OF OCCUPATION REQUIRING YOU TO LIFT HEAVY THINGS OR PUT YOUR BODY THROUGH A RANGE OF SWINGING, HANGING, PUSHING, AND PULLING MOVEMENTS, YOU'RE GOING TO HAVE TO DO STRENGTH

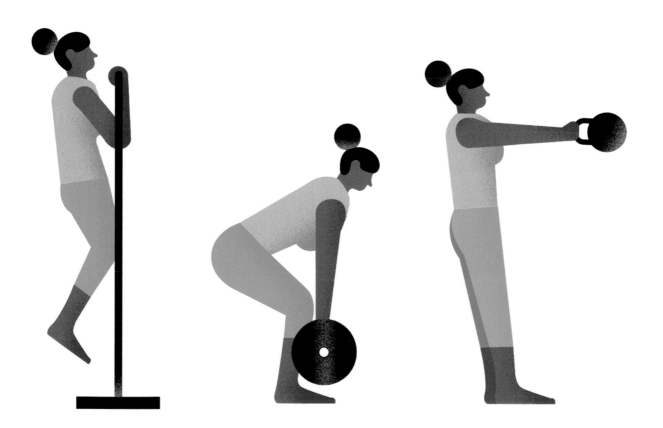

TRAINING. STRONGMAN ICON PAVEL TSATSOULINE (the man who brought kettlebells to the U.S.) called strength "the mother of all physical qualities." It is different from general cardiovascular fitness and flexibility, the two things that most exercisers target.

The definition of strength, in simplest terms, is the ability to carry a load from point A to point B. (When you can do that with speed, it's called power.) It requires having the structural ability in your muscles, tendons, and ligaments to meet the demands and carry the loads of life, and healthy-enough joints to support those loaded movements. Think of strength as physical integrity: the ability to handle everything life throws at you. Whether that's carrying three bags of groceries and a squirming child, moving your couch, or simply moving your own body weight through space, the requirement is the same: You want quality muscle tissue and resilient connective tissue. Cultivating strength is key to protecting yourself against injury, especially as you get older (you lose muscle mass as you age, so building it up while you still can preempts excessive loss). It's also key to avoiding much of the pain that accrues from daily life and engendering a positive and confident state of mind, not least because you look better, but also because strength training boosts mood-enhancing endorphins.

When you have a safe and effective strength-training program established—this may just include very short sessions, a couple times a week—you will also reduce the risk factors for diabetes (resistance training is shown to help prevent insulin resistance), heart disease, and cancer.

But how do you start? The options are multiple—weightlifting, kettlebells, bodyweight training—but they can be intimidating. Or they're not intimidating *enough*: Rushing into strength training from an unconditioned state, or doing it on your own without learning proper technique, is the fastest way to put wear and tear on the body. It puts strength on top of dysfunction because your joints and connective tissues are not ready for the load you ask them to carry, and if that happens, the physical therapist (or surgeon!) gets to see the consequences.

If you have access to a qualified trainer who can slowly ramp you up on a strength-training program, that's a great way to go. (Be picky—always get referrals.) For everyone else, there are ways to chart your own course.

I asked our Be Well strength coach and movement education trainer **Adam Ticknor** to map out a safe and effective arc for building strength step by step, from the ground up.

MONTH ONE Start with basic conditioning drills. Every day, do the following sequence five or six times throughout the day to build good movement patterns, turn on your trunk muscles, and prepare your shoulders, hips, and connective tissue. You can do it once when you get out of bed, and once after brushing your teeth after breakfast—that's two times before you even leave the house. Do it again instead of a midmorning coffee break; that's three. And so on.

HANG FOR 30 SECONDS. Use a pull-up bar installed in a doorway or a monkey bar in a local park. If you're in an office without access to a bar, do a modified body row using your desk or other sturdy table at your workplace: Sit on the floor with your legs extended all the way under the desk, grab on to the top of the desk, and, keeping your trunk tight and your body in a straight line or "plank," pull your chest up to the desk and hold that position for 30 seconds.

SQUAT FOR 30 SECONDS. With your feet hip-distance or wider, shins 90 degrees to the floor, reach your butt back as you squat as low as you can go without compromising shin position or letting your knees fall inward.

BEAR CRAWL FOR 30 SECONDS. Start on all fours with your hands on the floor, arms straight below your shoulders, knees beneath your hips and bent to ninety degrees, and feet raised so you're on your toes. Crawl forward across the room, then backward to starting position, moving the opposite hand and foot in unison: right hand and left foot move forward or backward at the same time, then the left hand and right foot. Keep your back flat, not rounded, as you crawl.

HANDSTAND AGAINST A WALL FOR 30 SECONDS. If getting vertical is too hard, walk your legs up a wall to 90 degrees or place your legs on a chair.

ADD A LOADED WALK (page 125), daily if you can.

As you're doing this, simultaneously train your sleep patterns—you'll need sleep as a foundation to gaining strength.

>>

Cultivating strength is key to protecting yourself against injury, especially as you get older.

<<

MONTH TWO Introduce a barbell deadlift with excellent technique (follow guidance and instructions on page 132). This one basic movement will give you a baseline of trunk and pelvic floor strength, correct knee and hip hinge movements, and get you to pull your shoulder into place before you use kettlebells. Keep doing your daily drills—you can vary it if you get comfortable. Keep doing your loaded walks.

MONTH THREE Introduce a basic two-arm kettlebell swing (to chest or nose height, not overhead). Group classes or online coaching can make this affordable—look for Russian-style kettlebell training. This puts what you've learned with the deadlift into dynamic motion. Start with a weight of 25 to 28 pounds for women or 30 to 40 pounds for men. Your aim: 100 swings a day, broken up through the day however you like. By the end of the month, it should only take three sets to achieve that 100-swing goal. Keep doing your deadlifts and daily loaded walk.

To successfully get strong requires ongoing development of skills and capacity—or your body adapts to the inputs and gets efficient with its muscle building, and you begin to plateau (not to mention get bored). These drills serve as your launching pad for a strength-building journey, so now go have fun! After three months of groundwork, you will be in great shape to join whatever strength and conditioning program appeals to you, whether it be barbell-oriented (Olympic lifting), kettlebell training, or calisthenics-based bodyweight training, or activities like rock climbing that build strength through motion. You are also prepped to do high-intensity metabolic workouts with much less risk of injury.

Strongfirst.com will connect you to expertly trained strength coaches.

THE LAZY, **LOADED WALK**

TAKE A DAILY WALK WITH A LITTLE LOAD ADDED TO YOUR BODY IN THE FORM OF A WEIGHTED VEST. THIS IS A SAFE, EFFECTIVE WAY TO CONDITION YOURSELF, BECAUSE IT LOADS THE SPINE FROM ALL DIRECTIONS WHILE COMPRESSING YOUR TRUNK, WHICH GIVES YOU STABILITY AS YOU MOVE AND IMPROVES YOUR POSTURE.

IT HELPS THE OVERUSED TRAPEZIUS MUSCLES (USED to carry your head) to release, and cues the entire trunk to "fire up" and hold you up straight. Loaded walking even helps free up the hip muscles, improving the hips' range of motion and thereby your gait.

The best way to do this is with a vest that distributes weight evenly around your torso. If you can, walk with a vest weighing no more than 10 percent of your body weight for about 45 minutes to an hour, daily or as often

as possible. (Don't run—it's too much impact!) You can hack this by wearing a loaded backpack on your front *and* your back, or a child in a carrier plus a backpack, but a vest is a lot easier. Get a vest that fits comfortably snug to your body, and if you have an injury, get evaluated by a professional first so you don't do any further damage.

There's no need to walk at a speedy clip; the idea is *long, lazy, and loaded.*

Moving improves everything:
your metabolism and your microbiome,
your sleep and all your body rhythms,
your immunity, your stress response,
and the overall balance in your life.

DITCH THE CHAIR (AND BREAK UP
YOUR BODY PATTERNS)

IT'S BEEN SAID THAT CHAIRS ARE JUNK FOOD FOR THE BODY. THAT MAY SOUND EXTREME BECAUSE THEY DO SERVE A USEFUL PURPOSE, BUT THE POINT IS TAKEN: THE EVER-PRESENT CHAIR (DESK, CAR, LIVING ROOM, DINING ROOM) HAS A SNEAKY WAY OF GETTING YOU INTO BAD HABITS WHILE ENGENDERING SOME DEGENER-

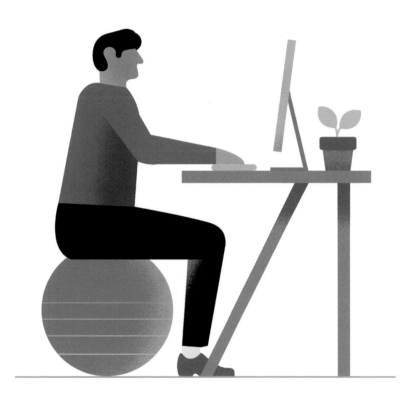

ATIVE TIVE SIDE EFFECTS. SEDENTARY LIFE ENCOURAGES a kind of physical atrophy—decline from disuse. When we are sitting, we are not moving. And we quite literally get stuck. The top conditioning coaches say that most modern adults have severe compromises in their mobility: Joints don't move smoothly and muscles don't fire easily in the ways that nature intended. Shoulders are locked, hips are frozen, elbows and forearms are constrained, and calves are tight. Meanwhile, the core and glute muscles get weak

and the back gets overstretched in a hunch. All this from sitting down for too much of the day! Try this drill: If you've been sitting at a desk for a couple of hours, stand up, then lower yourself to a sitting position on the floor (assuming you are injury-free, of course). Chances are this motion, which is a basic human function, is more creaky than fluid. But it shouldn't be. Sitting down on the floor and standing up is an important full-range-of-motion movement that keeps joints juicy while building functional muscle strength.

Become less attached to your chair (pun intended). Seek postural change throughout the day, and find opportunities to get low, stand back up, and move from side to side. It's not all-or-nothing here, because standing 100 percent of the time isn't ideal, either. Your body likes a multidimensional approach, involving different directions and planes.

HERE ARE 8 REMEDIES FOR SEDENTARY LIVING:

1. **IF YOUR DAILY LIFE INVOLVES SITTING, USE AN ERGONOMIC CHAIR.** My favorite ones allow movement as you sit, from the top-of-the-line Swopper stool to a large exercise ball (sized to allow you to keep your thighs parallel to floor with flat feet). These seats engage your core, keep your circulation going, and enliven your nervous system because you have to make constant micro movements to maintain your posture. If you don't have knee issues, an alternative is a kneeling chair. If you need back support, a good chiropractor should be able to advise the best option for you.

2. **IF USING AN EXERCISE BALL,** make sure to get a burst-proof ball that won't pop, and be cautious of it rolling out from under you if you sit down quickly (high heels can make this a liability). More stable versions of this include balls set into frames.

3. **ALTERNATE BETWEEN YOUR BALL AND A REGULAR CHAIR** until you are used to it—but don't stay sedentary! You still need to get up and move—take a stroll, do some stretches or lunges—at least every 45 minutes. Set a timer on your phone (or an old-fashioned sand hourglass) to sync you to this "Get up!" rhythm.

4. **INVEST IN AN ADJUSTABLE-HEIGHT OR SIT-TO-STAND DESK.** Tell your employer that these can boost productivity because the brain is more oxygenated, which gives you more mental energy, and focus increases as discomfort diminishes. A cheaper hack is a platform that goes on your existing desk to raise the height of a laptop, but the ideal setup lets you alternate sitting and standing. (For a mobility drill you can do while working at your computer, see howtobewell.com.)

5. **IF YOU CAN, CHANGE YOUR POSITIONS THROUGHOUT THE DAY.** Mix in periods of kneeling at a low table, sitting on the floor, and walking while you talk. This will completely transform the way you feel at the end of the day.

6. **IF YOU WEAR HEELS, TAKE THEM OFF AT YOUR DESK.** Sitting in them shortens the tendons of the leg. It's a prime cause of Achilles injuries for those who go straight from sitting to after-work running. It also helps to alternate days when you wear heels with days when you wear flats.

7. **NORMALIZE MOVING AT YOUR WORKPLACE.** This may seem intimidating, but why worry what your coworkers think? Keep *yourself* resilient and happy. Your outlier actions will probably start a trend toward a less static office culture. Try it and see!

8. **CONTINUE THIS PRIMAL MINDSET AT HOME.** Before plopping on the couch or chair, consider an alternative that forces you to use your body's full range of motion. Get down onto the ground to play with kids or pets, or to read. Some nights, eat dinner at a coffee table, seated on pillows. You could even swap out your couch for beanbags—getting in and out of those requires core and glute engagement. One of my favorite hacks: Store frequently used kitchen gear like plates and cups in a low cupboard. It forces you to squat down and stand up several times a day (squatting, not bending at the waist, gives you the benefits). And why not pull out your dustpan and brush instead of the vacuum so you get down low to clean your corners? Small changes like these make you use all of your body, more of the time.

CORRECT THE TECH INJURIES

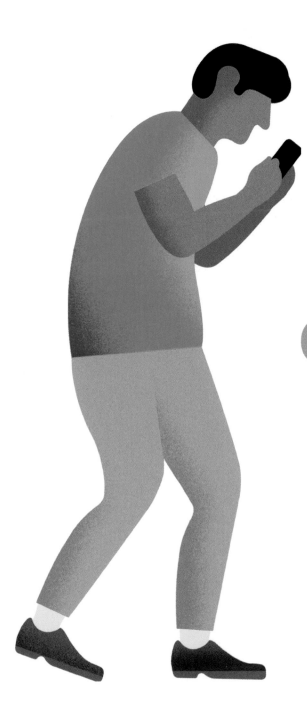

THERE'S A CLASS OF PHYSICAL COMPLAINTS THAT chiropractors and alignment experts call "tech injuries," and they are on the rise. These come from the small postural compromises we unconsciously make all day long from being tethered to computers and devices. These rolled or jutted-forward body shapes we fall into—sometimes for hours!—get repeated until they start pulling the spine out of alignment. This causes structural issues like back pain and hip imbalance and can also cause problems body-wide, because the nerve roots that run through the spinal canal, sending information throughout the nervous system, get pressured and cause localized dysfunctions. Headaches, digestive problems, and even fertility problems (and more) can be the unfortunate results.

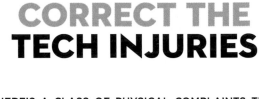

It can take a lot of effort, time, and money to undo spinal compromise, so don't let bad tech habits go uncorrected. **Dr. Keren Day,** the chiropractor and resident spinal expert at Be Well, explains how to avoid becoming her patient.

THE PROBLEM: THE FORWARD SLUMP

When you reach for a keyboard (or continuously hold a baby), your shoulders roll forward and your spine rounds. Your back is put into a negative stretch while the front of your body gets knotted from compression, causing back pain. (Did you know that tight muscles in your torso and belly can pull your spine out of line?) Oxygen flow is diminished, causing low energy and foggy thinking. The forward slump can even lead to a negative outlook—it is a posture of defeat. Plus, if you go from sitting in this forward roll position to pressing weights overhead during a workout, tendonitis or a torn rotator cuff can be the unintended consequence.

THE ANTIDOTE: Improve the ergonomics of your work-station. Your feet should be flat on the floor, your thighs parallel to the ground (raise on a footrest if needed), your elbows close to the body, and your forearms and hands parallel to the desktop with no unnatural raising of the wrists to meet the keyboard.

Invest in an ergonomic chair that supports the natural curve of the spine and avoids spinal compromises, and follow the 45-minute "Get up!" rule (page 127).

Shrug and rotate your shoulders frequently with shoulder shrugs and big circles of the arms.

Nightly, do chest- and back-opening postures such as restorative yoga poses like the reclining cross-legged pose (page 206), or the foam roller back opener sequence (page 139).

Do back and shoulder mobility exercises using our demo videos on howtobewell.com.

THE PROBLEM: TEXT NECK

This is a common misalignment of the handheld-gadget generation. Your neck juts forward as your eyes gaze at a device that's held out in front of you or low down. Squinting to read an overly small font causes the same effect—you tend to jut your head forward to read. If you chronically look down, you will overstretch the back of the neck—and possibly cut off your breath, too. Tension headaches and migraines can ensue; so can tennis elbow, carpal tunnel syndrome, numb or tingling arms, pain between shoulder blades, and shoulder tendonitis.

THE ANTIDOTE: Maintain an eye-level gaze no matter the device and ensure the font size is large enough to see easily. Never hold phones and tablets at lap level. Not only is it terrible for your reproductive system to have wire-less devices anywhere near your lap, it angles your chin down and strains the neck. Practice holding them at eye level as you type, or use your phone's dictation tool for texting. This spares your wrists and forearms unneeded

stress. It may take a day or two to master, but after that it's smooth sailing. If traveling by air, put your phone or tablet on a stand on the tray table while reading or view-ing media. When you're a passenger in a train or car, prop a small travel pillow under your elbow on the armrest to help you hold your device higher.

At your desk, ensure the center of your screen is at eye level whether you are sitting or standing. If you use a laptop, raise it on a platform—or even a big pile of books!—then accessorize with an external keyboard and an ergonomic mouse (which will counter any over-rotation of the wrist).

For both issues, practice the habit of bringing awareness to your body posture throughout the day. Notice if you are holding your breath, which further constricts the spine. Unfreeze yourself through conscious breathing, frequent movement, and making subtle adjustments as needed.

These repeated rolled or jutted-forward body shapes we fall into eventually can pull the spine out of alignment.

GET HIP ABOUT HIIT

HIIT IS HOT. HIGH-INTENSITY INTERVAL TRAINING (HITT) IS A QUICK, EFFICIENT WAY TO CONDITION YOUR BODY THROUGH SHORT BURSTS OF EXERCISE ALTERNATED WITH SLOWER RECOVERY SEGMENTS. IT IS A POW-ERFUL WAY TO REV YOUR FAT-BURNING METABOLISM, BUILD GLUCOSE TOLERANCE, AND BOOST COGNITIVE

FUNCTION (THANKS TO A SURGE OF A PROTEIN CALLED brain-derived neurotrophic factor). Studies show that HIIT is a more efficient way to achieve all these things than long, slow cardio workouts. While it's improving your cardiovascular health, pushing hard and fast for supershort bursts is also increasing your resting metabolism—you actually burn more energy in the 24 hours that follow—by spiking the hormones that burn fat and boosting the ability of the mitochondria to generate energy (which is important because mitochondrial function declines with age). It's also been shown that brief, very intense HIIT sessions improve insulin sensitivity for up to three days afterward. Bonus: HIIT can be done with minimal equipment; a speed rope or just your bodyweight will do.

If short and savage sounds better than an hour spent plodding on a stationary bike, note there are two caveats to this trend. First, HIIT is supposed to be masochistic. The bursts should feel grueling, close to your very max of effort (the point where talking is impossible). Second, it's important to first become conditioned and practice proper movement patterns (use the hang, squat, crawl sequence on page 123). If you increase intensity and speed *without* this foundation—say, by jumping into endless rounds of burpees without any prep—the odds of hurting yourself skyrocket. It's wise to ask yourself if you have established a good base of conditioning: Can you do five great chest-to-ground push-ups or one clean pull-up? You're cleared to go. (Third caveat for those with blood pressure or heart issues: Check in with your health professional about HIIT before doing it.)

Gradually scale your way up to the HIIT habit using these three protocols designed by HTBW pro Adam Ticknor. They keep the "high-intensity" part short and the "recovery" phase long—and will still get you the results you seek. In

each case, do several minutes of warming up (walking and mobility) first.

1. **FIND A VERY STEEP HILL.** Sprint up it as hard as you can for maximum 10 to 14 seconds. Rest for a full 3 minutes, walking lazily back down the hill. Repeat 7 times.

2. **ON A STATIONARY BIKE OR ROWING MACHINE** set to moderate resistance, do a 20-second high-intensity sprint, followed by 2 to 3 minutes mellow peddling or rowing. Repeat 6 to 8 times. Check out some online training videos for good rowing form.

3. **USING A JUMP ROPE,** build your way up to what are called double-unders (where the rope passes under your feet two times for each jump). This builds terrific core stability, and learning its novel movement pattern strengthens brain function, too.

Until you can perform successive double-unders, your workout will be: Warm up for several minutes doing single-under jumps, with 25 attempts at the double-under. Then, for 2 minutes without stopping, do *as many rounds as possible* of 30 seconds of single-unders followed by 5 sit-ups, then pick one of the following and complete 5 reps: pull-ups, pushups, or dips. Rest for 2 minutes. Repeat this 3 to 5 times. Increase the workout window to 3 minutes when you are able.

Once you have mastered double-unders, change the first step above to *as many rounds as possible* of 25 double-unders.

MORNING MOBILITY DRILL

DO THE FOLLOWING FIVE-MINUTE MOBILITY DRILL IN THE MORNING BEFORE YOU GET OUT OF BED. IT WILL "PRIME THE PUMP" FOR THE DAY AHEAD, ENSURING YOUR JOINTS MOVE FLUIDLY AND COUNTERING STIFFNESS AND SORENESS. BASICALLY, IT REMINDS YOUR BODY HOW TO MOVE AFTER A NIGHT OF LYING DOWN. TRY IT FOR A WEEK

AND SEE IF YOUR MOVEMENT THROUGHOUT THE DAY—and any workout you do later—feels smoother and more comfortable. Do the moves lying down on your back, in any order you like, repeating each movement 10 times.

ARMS

WRIST ROLLS: Raise your arms straight toward the ceiling. Roll your wrists in circles, clockwise and counterclockwise.

SCAPULAR SHRUGS: Raise your arms straight toward the ceiling, elbows locked. Push upward so your scapula (shoulder blades) rise off the bed, then release.

OVERHEAD REACHES: Raise your arms straight toward the ceiling, palms facing up and fingers interlaced. Reach your hands as high and as far back toward the headboard or wall behind you as possible. Return to the starting position and repeat.

REACH AND PULSE: With your hands on the headboard or wall behind you, push in pulses while pressing the small of your back into the mattress.

PRAYER STRETCH: Clasping your hands in front of your face, with your elbows and forearms glued together at 90 degrees to your torso, reach your hands over and behind you to the back wall. Then return them in front of you and, with your elbows at your belly button, stretch clasped hands towards your feet, forearms still glued together. This should be one smooth movement. In Prayer Pose, do Wrist Rolls, clockwise and counterclockwise.

FOREARM CIRCLES: Extend one arm straight above the shoulder. Keeping the arm locked straight and upper arm stationary, circle the forearm in big circles, aiming to get your thumb close to your bicep. Repeat with your other arm.

LEGS

ANKLE ROLLS: Start with your legs straight and relaxed. Make big circles with your feet, clockwise and counterclockwise.

POINT AND FLEX: Start with your legs straight and relaxed. Point your toes to the bed then flex the foot the opposite way. (You can do both feet at once.)

KNEE CIRCLES: Start with your legs straight and relaxed. Lift one knee up to 90 degrees and circle your foot in the air, drawing a big radius with your toe, clockwise and counterclockwise. Repeat with your other leg.

HIP SWIVELS: Bend your legs and place your feet hip-distance apart, halfway to your hips. Swivel your hips from side to side, allowing your knee to fall toward your opposite heel.

EGGBEATERS: Do Knee Circles with both legs at once, feeling the movement in your hips.

HEAD AND NECK

CHIN TO CHEST: Tuck your chin inward, stretching the back of your neck.

CHIN-UPS: Keeping your head flat and looking at the ceiling, reach your face upward to the ceiling, lifting your neck off the bed.

SIDE TO SIDE: Shake your head "no."

EAR TO SHOULDER: Stretch your right ear to your right shoulder, stretching the left side of your neck. Switch sides.

THE SINGLE BEST MOVE: THE DEADLIFT

IF YOU HAD TO PICK A SINGLE FITNESS MOVEMENT TO KEEP YOU STRONG AND HEALTHY FOR LIFE, THE BAR-BELL DEADLIFT SHOULD BE IT. THIS CLASSIC WEIGHTLIFTING MOVE INVOLVES HINGING FORWARD AT THE HIPS TO GRASP A HEAVILY LOADED BARBELL, HINGING STRAIGHT UP TO STANDING, PULLING THE BARBELL TO

KNEE HEIGHT, AND THEN LOWERING THE BARBELL again. Done correctly, this supersimple movement is incredibly high-yield: As a compound movement that requires multiple major muscle groups to work together, it fires up every muscle in your body and builds healthy muscle tissue from top to toe. A deadlift demands powerful trunk contraction and pelvic floor stability, which together build a healthy core and a strong, resilient back. It develops the (typically underused) glutes and hamstrings, activating the body's main source of power. It enhances blood flow to all the tissues, which, combined with that better pelvic condition, brings benefits for sex—yes, deadlifts can help spark your orgasmic potential. And it's not just for heavyweight bodybuilders! It can be safely learned by anyone—assuming you are starting without injury—and scaled up gradually as your capacity grows.

To learn it, once you've done several weeks of basic strength conditioning (page 122), a few sessions with a coach is best. (These days, you can even ask coaches for online reviews of your form.) Start with a bar loaded way beyond what you can lift and have a coach check your hinging motion—this will teach you to tighten your trunk and load your body before you accelerate, and it will engrain the proper mechanics of movement. Once you're ready to start lifting, load a bar with weight below your bodyweight and do single lifts with 1-minute rests in between. Then, over the next two weeks, increase the load to your bodyweight, and then, over the two weeks following that, to 125 percent of your bodyweight. As you increase the weight, *gradually* increase the number of sets, to 5 sets of 5 lifts in a workout.

The book *Starting Strength* by Mark Rippetoe includes an excellent primer for the deadlift.

Done correctly, this supersimple movement fires up every muscle in your body and builds healthy muscle tissue from top to toe.

BECOME A
BETTER RUNNER

RUN LIKE THE WIND—BUT LEARN HOW TO DO IT FIRST. IT SOUNDS RIDICULOUS TO SUGGEST THAT YOU'D HAVE TO *LEARN* TO RUN. AFTER ALL, YOU'VE BEEN RUNNING ALMOST SINCE YOU STARTED WALKING. BUT IT'S ACTUALLY A TECHNICAL SKILL THAT REQUIRES DEVELOPING AND HONING BECAUSE OTHERWISE, BAD FORM CAN

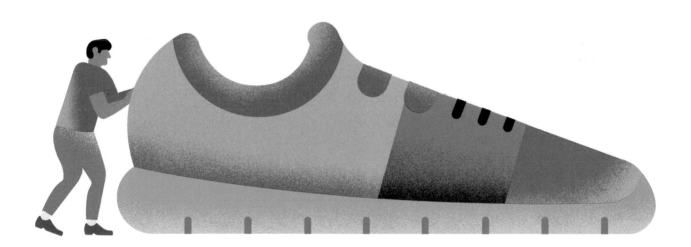

TAKE YOU DOWN. THE NUMBER OF PATIENTS I SEE with an impact-related injury has made me skeptical of the sport—I've always felt it's fantastic for the head but not so good for the body, because constant running practice tends to put far too much pressure on the joints. But the proper skills can totally change the game and teach you proper alignment. Running training programs like Chi Running and the Pose Method can teach you to strike the ground with your foot directly under your pelvis instead of out front (which makes you "brake" and jar your body with each step), to position your torso correctly, and to strike the ground at a much quicker and more efficient

tempo. (Whichever way you go, be cautious of treadmill running; it's one of the main ways you can get into bad "striking patterns" and reinforce bad habits.) With practice, you'll begin to move effectively and fluidly, starting to run farther and faster than before.

Safer ways to get your cardiovascular training in at the gym and that use more of your body are a rowing machine or the angled, non-mechanized Jacob's Ladder, which puts your body through a full range of motion while only moving as fast as you can move. A stationary bike is another safe option but it doesn't give the same full-body movement.

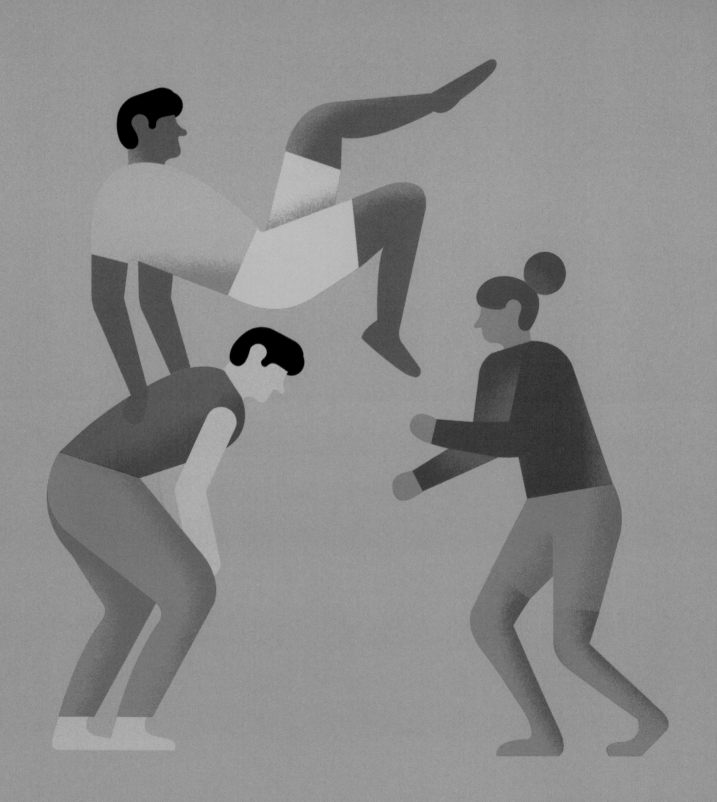

PLAY LIKE **A CHILD**

WHAT'S THE GOAL OF EXERCISE? IS IT TO MAKE THE BEST SCORES AND THE BEST GAINS, TO BEAT THE COM-PETITION? OR IS IT TO BE THE BEST *YOU*: A CURIOUS AND ENGAGED HUMAN ANIMAL, FREE TO MOVE THROUGH THE WORLD IN A WAY THAT MAKES YOU FEEL THE MOST ALIVE? THE LATTER IS WHAT YOU ACHIEVE

WHEN YOU STEP BEYOND LINEAR INDOOR WORK-outs and into nature's playground, moving through, over, under, and around its organic features just like you did when you were a child. When was the last time you broke up your run by, say, climbing a tree trunk, hopping over boulders, long-jumping across a lawn, or hanging from a branch? Or turned your everyday hike into an off-road adventure, rock-hopping across rivers and squeezing through fences?

Something amazing happens when you let yourself play: More of your body wakes up. Physically, when you jump, land, and mix up angles of movement, the mechano-receptors in your muscle tendon junctions, bones, and ligaments activate and help you determine where you are in space, making you agile (and less prone to injury should you stumble or fall during everyday activities). When you solve the physical challenge of how to get from here to there by trying new body shapes and making quadrupedal movements, your brain fires up to solve spatial problems and your body connects more deeply

with your mind. You might enter the flow state—fully present in the moment. When you make physical contact with nature's unpredictable terrain, you even have to face fear—this builds resilience against stress. Plus, as any kid knows, play is fun—and free!

Start by simply looking around you next time you're hiking or running, even in an urban park. Look to the side of the trail: What's there to play on? (If you're with kids, this will come easy; park benches and walls count, too.) Explore the feature, get on it, get off it, hang from it, and test it.

A FEW OF MY FAVORITE PRIMAL PLAY RESOURCES:

- MoveNat (movnat.com)
- Animal Flow (animalflow.com)
- Peace Sticks (peacesticks.com)

Something amazing happens when you let yourself play: More of your body wakes up.

BALANCE THE YANG WITH THE YIN:
REST AND RECOVERY

WE ARE A CULTURE OF EXTREMES. WE EITHER DO NOT MOVE AND EXERCISE ENOUGH OR WE HIT THE GYM INTENSELY, TO THE POINT WHERE INJURY CAN OFTEN OCCUR. IT'S THE MODERN POLARITY—WE'RE EITHER UNDERACTIVE OR OVERACTIVE—BUT WHAT WOULD SERVE US BEST IS TO FIND THE FUSION OF THE TWO EXTREMES AND BALANCE EFFORT WITH REST.

Rest and recovery is a nonnegotiable part of any training protocol. However, this message has gotten diminished in our achievement-obsessed, goal-oriented culture, where we often rush to tough spin classes multiple times per week or sign up for intense training schedules that promise the world if we do them hard enough. Sometimes the motivation is a personal goal, like getting in shape for a big event; often, if we tune in to the *why*, it's because intense physical effort is the one thing that dispels the anxiety and intensity of our lives, and helps us feel grounded and present.

None of these are negative reasons to work out, of course, but for the sake of longevity—and making gains to feel really good about—it is wise to pause and assess if your training has too much fiery and aggressive yang and not enough restorative and healing yin. Just as racecars break down more often and spend more time in the shop, if you are an intense, "type A" exerciser who loves fast and forceful workouts, you need to treat your vehicle with grade-A care and know that the harder you train, the more important recovery time becomes. That doesn't mean becoming a couch potato on your days off. Instead, gentler forms of active recovery like long, lazy, loaded walks (page 125), mobility and skills practice work (like mastering a perfect handstand), walking and playing freely outside with no goal in mind, or doing a complementary type of practice like tai chi, qigong, or yoga (a restorative kind, not an ultra-demanding kind) provide a quieter and restorative yin-like balance to all that muscle-burning, yang-like activity. So does foam rolling (page 137) and dynamic stretching, which stretches muscles safely and effectively

through a full range of movement—the opposite of the old-school approach of holding a static stretch until it hurts, which can cause tearing at the muscle insertion points. This technique is easy to learn and practice. And don't forget sleep—a nonnegotiable recovery method for anyone who trains hard.

Light-intensity exercise promotes blood flow and helps clear the lactic acid byproduct of intense exercise, which, if not flushed out, will limit muscle tissues' function and make your next training session harder. It can help prevent extreme soreness and ensure mobility is maintained. Proper rest lets the body divert resources to healing and restoration, and adapt to the effects of the training you've just done. It also ensures that you develop the complementary aspect of your fitness protocol: an ability to tune in to your body and notice where it needs support, as well as a higher awareness of how your body moves, which can support any kind of movement practice you do. If you're an alpha-type exerciser, be sure to include some counterbalancing practices into your week to achieve a more harmonized approach to your total fitness.

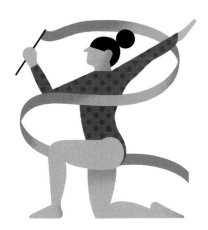

ROLL YOUR **FASCIA**

FIVE TO TEN MINUTES A DAY ON A FOAM ROLLER WORKS WONDERS FOR YOUR BODY. CONSIDER THE ROLLER A SURVIVAL TOOL FOR MODERN LIFE: AN ANTIDOTE TO SEDENTARY LIVING THAT ALLOWS YOU TO MASSAGE MUSCLES AND TENDONS THAT YOUR HANDS COULD NEVER REACH AND TO DECOMPRESS YOUR SPINE AFTER

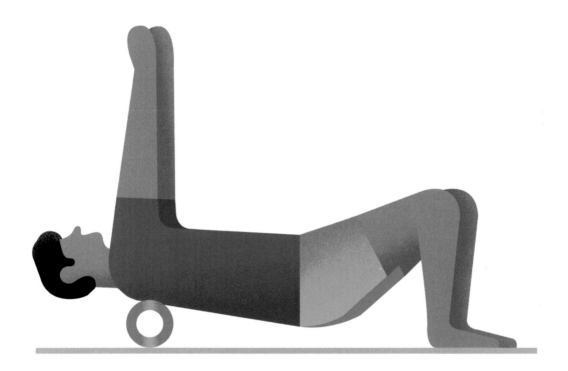

SITTING. IT'S ALSO A DIY WAY TO GET CIRCULATION and healing going in sore muscles after hard workouts and an almost-instant energy reviver, because as circulation increases and sore muscles release, oxygen flow to the brain is boosted. This inexpensive thirty-six-inch-long cylinder can turn you into your own bodyworker!

One reason that foam rolling is so powerful is that it stimulates and smoothes a type of connective tissue that is rarely acknowledged by Western medicine: the fascia. Your fascia is a thin, gelatinous membrane that surrounds and

is fused with the bones, muscles, tendons, nerves, blood vessels, and organs in your body. In Latin, the word translates as "band," which describes the appearance of these continuous sheets of soft tissue. Superficial fascia lies just beneath your skin. Deep fascia is slightly tougher and more compact. It supports, connects, and compartmentalizes the different body parts and is especially enmeshed within the muscular system.

The fascia enables the forces of the muscles to be transmitted safely and effectively without harming the other tissues. It helps muscles to change shape and length during movement and therefore ensures proper alignment. I believe it is also the medium for the energy meridians known to Chinese medicine. From the Western point of view, the fascia is now being called a sensory organ because it's where the nerves sit and where pain originates and is communicated to the brain.

HOW TO BE WELL EXPERT Body alignment expert **Lauren Roxburgh** is an authority on foam rolling and a friend of the Be Well team. She calls foam rolling an essential self-care tool in a world where we are "overworked, overstressed, overfed, and overstimulated."

In a healthy state your fascia will be smooth, flexible, and fluid. But because it is where many of us store stress, tension, and toxins, when the fascia becomes subject to inflammation or injuries, to poor posture and repetitive stress, or even to emotional trauma or fear, it can lose its suppleness and become thick and tight. Think of a sponge that has dried up and gotten all brittle and stiff: When you add water to the sponge, it becomes fluid and supple. Rolling your body out is effectively putting hydration and "juiciness," which are qualities we associate with youthfulness, back into the fascia, and it also boosts lymphatic drainage to flush toxins. This is incredibly self-healing and helps to reverse the energy-stagnating, pain-inducing toll of our sedentary modern lives.

Rolling regularly is key to enjoying the benefits. So is broadening your mindset: Use foam rolling as part of a wellness ritual, not just to target stiff muscles at the end of the day, but to help you destress, improve your digestion, and calm your nervous system. You can do this with simple ten-minute sequences that help you create balance and tone in your entire body from head to toe in an integrated way. They can be easily worked into everyday life, either after exercising or before bed.

>>

Movement causes muscle tissue to produce proteins called myokines that have important disease-preventive and anti-inflammation functions.

FOAM ROLLER BACK OPENER SEQUENCE

This helps get rid of kinks and knots from sitting and hunching forward, and it's also a stress reliever because the weight of the world often loads itself onto the shoulders and back. It helps wake you up, too—try it when you are stuck in a middle-of-the-day slump.

STEP 1   LIE ON YOUR BACK WITH BENT LEGS AND FEET HIP-WIDTH APART. PLACE YOUR FOAM roller horizontally beneath your middle back, and your hands behind your head, supporting its weight.

STEP 2   LIFT UP YOUR HIPS AND WALK YOUR FEET OUT ABOUT A FOOT. AS YOU INHALE, ROLL your body down the roller until your neck touches it; exhale as you roll it back to the middle of your back. As you do this, drive the movement with your legs, keep your core muscles engaged, and activate your thighs. Repeat the motion for 30 seconds to 1 minute. To vary the way the roller gets into your muscles, you can change the way your weight falls on it by reaching your arms behind you (so your elbows are in line with your ears) or extending your arms straight up to the ceiling.

STEP 3   LIE LENGTHWISE ON THE ROLLER WITH YOUR HEAD RESTING ON THE TOP END. BEND your knees with your feet on the floor, hip-width apart. Placing your hands at your ears, drop your elbows to the floor. Inhale and exhale, feeling your chest and shoulders open, for 30 seconds.

STEP 4   NEXT, GENTLY ROLL SIDE TO SIDE, LETTING THE ROLLER NUDGE AND MASSAGE THE space between your spine and shoulder blades for up to 1 minute. This gently decompresses the spine and helps create more space between the vertebrae. You may also feel more energized and awake afterward.

Visit howtobewell.com for how-to videos of Lauren's foam-rolling sequences.

HOW TO CHOOSE A ROLLER

Choose a medium-density roller with a little texture on its surface (the texture helps promote lymphatic drainage). It should have support but just a little give to it, too.

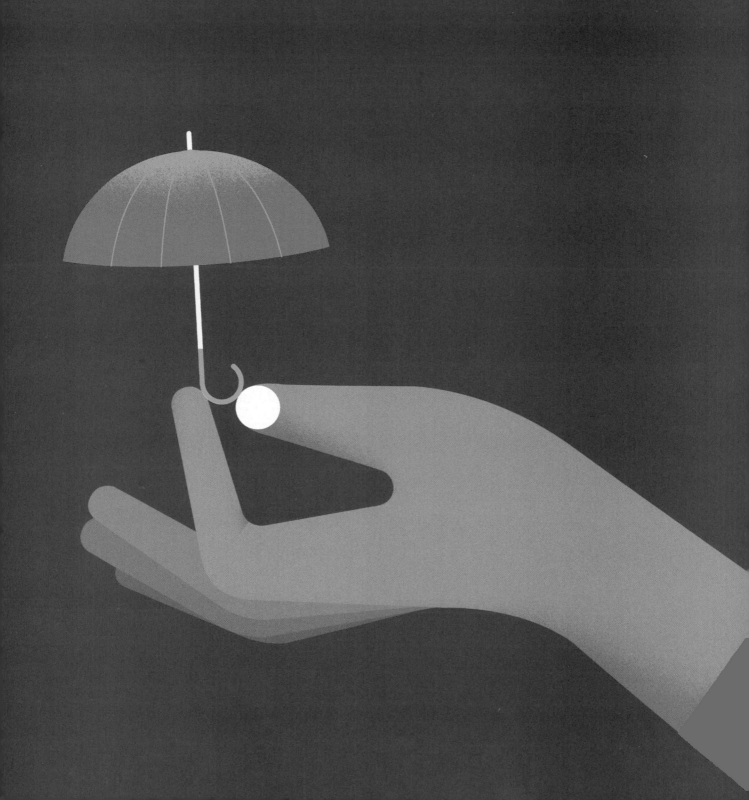

PROTECT

SO MANY OF THE INGREDIENTS IN THE PRODUCTS
we interact with very intimately each day—the things that
we eat, slather on ourselves, inhale, and sleep amid—are
unregulated by any authority. Thought "someone else"
would be ensuring that everything available to you is totally
safe? Think again. When it comes to protecting your health
and well-being, the investigating and governing body
is you!

We live with a sea of stressors that our ancestors could
never have anticipated and that our bodies did not evolve
to handle. It is overwhelming our detoxification systems,
which exist to clear as many toxins as possible but get
taxed to the max dealing with chemicals, carcinogenic
compounds, and even invisible electromagnetic frequencies. We are only just starting to understand the
impact of chronic exposure to these unnatural stressors,
but nobody is addressing how the individual elements
interact with each other in our bodies. What integrative
doctors do know is that chronic exposure to low-dose
chemicals almost certainly plays a role in the development of autoimmune diseases, cancer, neurological
diseases, fertility issues, ADHD, allergies, and more, and
their slow buildup can be the reason for all kinds of nag-
ging symptoms that we write off as the fatigue of modern
life or inevitable effects of aging.

Remove as many of the damaging influences as you can,
replace them with simple alternatives, and start to give
your body the conditions it needs to steadily do its work
of keeping you well. If you begin with one step today and
then another and so on, over time you will do a clean sweep.

AUDIT **YOUR MEDS**

SINCE WHEN DID IT BECOME COMMONPLACE TO WALK AWAY FROM DOCTORS' VISITS WITH A PRESCRIPTION (OR TWO, OR THREE) IN HAND? THE LAST TWO DECADES OR SO. OUR FRACTURED AND OVERTAXED MEDICAL SYSTEM HAS BECOME FOCUSED ON FIXING SYMPTOMS AS FAST AS POSSIBLE USING PHARMACEUTICAL

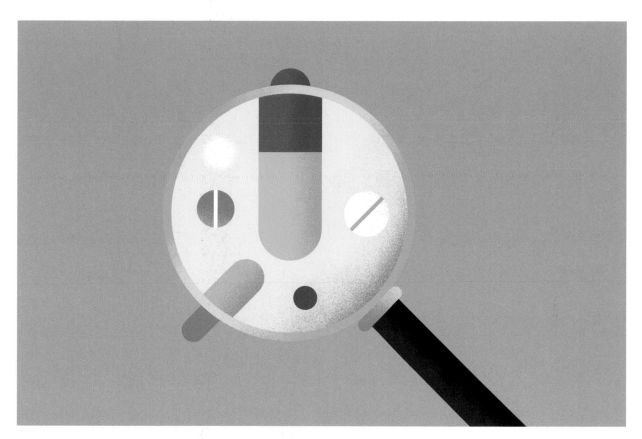

MEDICATIONS—WITH BARELY A NOD AT THE MANY side effects and frequent ineffectiveness of this strategy (which often doesn't resolve the actual underlying issues). This speed- and profit-driven approach is starting to catch up with us.

I'm seeing a sharp increase in the number of young patients suffering from autoimmune diseases like lupus, Hashimoto's disease, and Crohn's disease. Often, rounds of prescription antibiotics, prescribed for acne, sinus issues, or minor childhood ailments, combined with poor diet, are at the root of these conditions and have caused the gut to become damaged and inflamed. A process of gut repair and restoration is what's required (page 174), not just more symptom-reducing drugs. On top of this, prescriptions for sleep-aid drugs (which don't tend to restore proper sleep patterns for the long term) are common. Antidepressants are also dispensed like candy and can cause weight gain, decreased libido and sexual dysfunction, and aggressive behavior or suicidal thoughts—and many experts are beginning to agree that they are sometimes more harmful than effective. This rampant prescribing is not as innocuous as it may seem. There is strong evidence that adverse effects of new drugs are kept hidden. A study published in a prestigious medical journal found that almost 65 percent of side effects found in drug trials are left out of the reports that doctors use to make treatment decisions. (The antibiotic group fluoroquinolones, which includes ciprofloxacin, is currently making waves for serious side effects.)

In my opinion, the three worst offenders among problem-causing prescription and over-the-counter drugs are proton pump inhibitors for acid reflux (because they cause an imbalance in the microbiome that creates a higher risk for infections and inhibits the absorption of nutrients, plus they may be connected to dementia and earlier death); anti-inflammatory drugs like ibuprofen and celecoxib (which can cause nausea, vomiting, stomach ulcers, damage to the intestinal lining and leaky gut, headaches, and dizziness); and statin drugs for managing cholesterol (which can cause memory and neurological problems and achy muscles, among other issues). Then there's the devastating addiction epidemic caused by the overprescription of opioid painkillers. These drugs are for the most part treating, and sometimes suppressing, symptoms, but not resolving the underlying cause of the problem. It's like seeing the oil light go on in your car, but instead of going to a mechanic for a look under the hood, you stick a Band-Aid over the light and keep driving. To make matters worse, you often end up taking multiple drugs to suppress a number of different symptoms because the problem just pops up in new locations, trying to alert you to an underlying issue.

How do *you* chart a course through our increasingly pharmaceutical-based health system to avoid taking unnecessary drugs and ensure you treat illnesses at their cause? It's a big question, but here's a basic primer:

1. **NEVER STOP TAKING A MEDICATION ON YOUR OWN,** but do an audit of any medications you are currently taking: Ask your provider why you are on them to evaluate whether they are essential, how they interact with your other medications, and whether alternative actions (particularly in diet and lifestyle) could take their place. (See 10 Questions, opposite.)

2. **LEARN ABOUT THE ROOT CAUSES** of, and successful rebalancing and repair strategies for, some of the most medicated conditions of today: inflammation, autoimmune issues, high cholesterol, anxiety and depression, skin and sinus issues, and frequent viruses and infections. With this knowledge, you can begin to look at prescribed medications with clearer eyes and make choices for strategies that deal with the underlying issues, either in tandem with medication or instead of it. To help you get started, the "What to Do When . . ." section on page 245 shares some basic protocols for common conditions.

3. **EDUCATE YOURSELF ON ALTERNATIVES,** using high-quality resources. If you can afford to see a functional medicine practitioner with a good reputation, this can be an excellent start; find one through functionalmedicine.org.

ASK YOUR DOCTOR THE "10 BIG QUESTIONS" ABOUT THE DRUGS YOU'VE BEEN PRESCRIBED

1. WHAT DOES THIS MEDICATION DO?

2. IS THIS DRUG INTENDED TO CURE MY UNDERLYING CONDITION or is it intended to give me relief from my symptoms?

3. WHAT ARE THE POTENTIAL NEGATIVE EFFECTS? Are they minor or major? Common or rare?

4. HAVE LONG-TERM STUDIES BEEN DONE ON THIS DRUG? Have studies been done for this drug on the elderly or women? (Be aware that many studies are conducted on young or middle-aged men, who often have different responses to medications and to dosages. Be especially sure to ask this question if you are going to take the drug long-term.)

5. DO THE BENEFITS OUTWEIGH THE RISKS?

6. IS THIS MEDICATION INTENDED TO PREVENT A PROBLEM OR TREAT ONE?

7. WHAT IS THE EVIDENCE THAT THIS DRUG IS ACTUALLY EFFECTIVE?

8. WHAT IS THE NNT (NUMBER NEEDED TO TREAT) FOR THIS MEDICATION? (You can look it up yourself on thennt.com, usually by drug category [statins] rather than brand name [Lipitor].)

9. ARE THERE NATURAL ALTERNATIVES I MIGHT TRY FIRST?

10. I'D LIKE TO TRY NATURAL ALTERNATIVES FIRST. Would you be willing to let me go that route for three months and then retest me?

There is strong evidence that adverse effects of new drugs are kept hidden.

THE BURDEN OF TOXINS: A DOCTOR'S MANIFESTO

FOLLOW THE PRECAUTIONARY PRINCIPLE:

IF SOMETHING IS NOT FULLY PROVEN SAFE, DON'T TAKE A CHANCE.

AVOID GMOS IN EVERYTHING YOU EAT.

THE ENVIRONMENT AROUND YOUR CELLS INFLUENCES WHETHER DISEASE-CAUSING GENES GET SWITCHED ON OR STAY OFF.

TOXINS AND POOR DIET CREATE ONE OF THE WORST ENVIRONMENTS POSSIBLE.

THE POWERS THAT BE WON'T DRIVE THE CHANGES WE NEED.

CONSUMER ACTION INFLUENCES THE MARKET. DEMAND CHANGES FROM MANUFACTURERS AND REGULATORY AGENCIES.

EDUCATE YOURSELF ABOUT EVERYDAY ENDOCRINE-DISRUPTING CHEMICALS

IN FOODS, COSMETICS, AND FURNISHINGS, WHICH WREAK HAVOC ON NORMAL HORMONE FUNCTION.

OTHERS MAY DISMISS YOUR EFFORTS TO REDUCE AND REPLACE THE TOXINS IN YOUR LIFE.

IGNORE THEM, FOLLOW YOUR INSTINCTS, AND CARRY ON.

FOCUS ON THE SMALL, PROACTIVE THINGS YOU CAN DO

INSTEAD OF WORRYING ABOUT ALL THAT YOU CANNOT. IT'S ABOUT GRADUALLY DECREASING YOUR TOXIC LOAD; ONE SMALL CHANGE WILL LEAD TO ANOTHER, AND THE BENEFITS WILL ADD UP.

CLEAN EATING CHEAT SHEET

SHIFTING TO TOXIN-FREE FOODS IS ONE OF THE MOST IMPORTANT THINGS YOU CAN DO FOR YOUR HEALTH. IT'S A WIN-WIN: IT REDUCES EXPOSURE TO CHEMICALS RESPONSIBLE FOR BEHAVIORAL, NEUROLOGICAL, AND AUTOIMMUNE DISORDERS AND RESPIRATORY DISEASES (AMONG OTHER THINGS) WHILE INCREASING THE

NUTRITIONAL VALUE OF THE FOODS YOU EAT. EVEN as I write, new information from Europe is alerting us that pesticides and other agricultural chemicals are more dangerous to the brain than we've been told—and especially hazardous to mothers-to-be and children. However, it's not always possible to do a clean sweep and go fully organic all at once, plus it can be confusing to navigate food groups like meat. Knowing where to start can feel overwhelming. Keep in mind that perfect is the enemy of good: Start with the items that you eat most frequently, and as other food products run out, replenish them with cleaner alternatives. Eating low on the food chain, with an abundance of vegetables supported by some healthy fats and small amounts of high-quality proteins, keeps things straightforward and affordable. And it bears repeating: Nonorganic processed foods are likely to be filled with chemical residues and genetically engineered ingredients like industrial seed oils and corn, soy, and beet-sugar products. Steer clear.

Use the following tips to guide your purchases. Start with what you can, and know that one small change, and then another, will transform your kitchen within a few months. The mantra is *Make progress—don't get paralyzed by perfection!*

FRESH PRODUCE

Not all produce is treated equally: Some fruits and vegetables are more likely to be sprayed with pesticides, herbicides, or fungicides, or are more easily penetrated by these chemicals. Some of the most likely contenders are berries, apples, spinach, grapes, potatoes, celery, and bell peppers. If you're on a budget, use the Environmental Working Group's Dirty Dozen and Clean Fifteen

lists to help you prioritize (also available as an app from ewg.org) and ensure the things you eat most are organic or have been sprayed with the least amount of chemicals. Shop at farmers' markets where you can learn which farms without organic certification follow safer, chemical-free practices—there are some—but be sure to quiz growers on what pesticides *and* herbicides they use (be skeptical if they claim not to use them but their produce is huge and abundant).

Check out whatsonmyfood.org to get a telling glimpse of the amounts of pesticide residues found on everyday foods—like a whopping sixty-eight types found on conventional cilantro—and why they are of concern.

DRIED GOODS: GRAINS, BEANS, LEGUMES

It's becoming common knowledge that conventional corn and soy products in the U.S. are almost all genetically engineered and of dubious safety—I recommend buying only organic versions of these foods. But the emerging issue of the antibiotic (and known carcinogenic) herbicide ingredient glyphosate has made a much bigger group of foods suspect, in particular crops like wheat, oats, beans, and lentils (see page 153). This is another very good reason to keep grain consumption low (or dialed down to zero!) and starchy beans and legumes at moderate levels. If you do use these foods, definitely make them organic. (See page 37 if you suspect you might have a problem digesting these foods due to their lectin content.)

Another new and growing concern is arsenic found in rice. Organic can't help you here, as this toxin—which is associated with heart disease and some cancers after long-term exposure to high levels—is absorbed from contaminated water and soil regardless of growing technique. Keep your intake of rice (and products made from it, including pastas, crackers, and milks) moderate, and cook in abundant water to reduce exposure (1 cup rice to 6 cups water; drain off excess). Soaking rice before cooking helps reduce the levels considerably. And don't overdo it on brown rice because it has the highest arsenic load. Instead, make cauliflower rice (page 63)!

ANIMAL PRODUCTS

Since toxins concentrate as you go higher up the food chain, sourcing cleaner animal products is extra important. Unfortunately, the majority of conventionally farmed meat, poultry, dairy products, and eggs contain antibiotics and hormones. An estimated 70 percent of antibiotics in the U.S. are used in animal agriculture, mainly to help animals grow faster and resist diseases caused by overcrowding.

MEAT: When we consume antibiotics in meat, they not only change the composition of our microbiome and may cause hormone issues (including early puberty in children), they also contribute to the collective problem of antibiotic resistance. Conventionally farmed animals are also almost always raised on genetically modified corn or soy feed, which is laced with pesticides and herbicides and high in inflammatory omega-6 fatty acids. By contrast, animal products from pastured or grass-fed animals that feast on leafy greens will be higher in health-protecting omega-3 fatty acids, cancer-fighting conjugated linoleic acid, and essential fat-soluble vitamins A, D, E, and K_2.

As you shop, keep asking what the animal your meat comes from eats, because that determines the level of nutrition and exposure to contamination that *you* get. That said, you need to ask the right questions. The term "grass-fed," for example, can be used by grain-fed feedlots that also use antibiotics, hormones, or pesticides, even if the animal has only eaten grass for a short period. Look for "100 percent grass-fed," and if it's also certified organic, all the better. Likewise, the term "pasture raised" has no common standard or requirement for verification, so look for an additional certification on the label, such as USDA Organic (for beef and dairy) or a Global Animal Partnership rating of Step 4 and above (for beef and pork). For a full list of food labels, visit the Consumer Reports website greenerchoices.org. (Note that "natural" on a meat label is not an indication of quality. It simply means the product contains no additives.)

The Global Animal Partnership is a nonprofit alliance of producers, retailers, animal advocates, and scientists dedicated to improving farm animal welfare and recognizing farmers and ranchers who exceed industry standards. Its five-step rating program, used by retailers like Whole Foods, can help you make more informed decisions about meat, poultry, eggs, and dairy.

RULE OF THUMB: Get the best meat you can afford, and if it's not 100 percent grass-fed, consume it in moderation.

POULTRY: Factory-farmed poultry is another sad and toxic story. In the U.S., chemical baths are often used to clean the processed birds, and phosphate, a vascular toxin banned in Europe, is often injected to boost plumpness and moisture. Whenever possible, source local, organic, and humanely and verified-pasture-raised birds. If this isn't possible, your second-best bet is organic poultry from a known supplier who air-chills instead of chemically bathes.

>> **When it comes to protecting your health and well-being, the investigating and governing body is you.** <<

DAIRY AND EGGS: If you choose to eat dairy, definitely choose organic, but be scrupulous about sources (check the Cornucopia Institute scorecard mentioned on page 48). For eggs, know that on their own, the terms "cage free," "free range," and "pasture raised" are no indicators of ethical treatment, healthy diet, or overall vital well-being for the hens. Look for a Certified Humane Raised & Handled label. Buying pastured eggs from local producers is best if within reach, but to rate your store-bought options, use Cornucopia's Organic Egg Scorecard.

FISH: Picking fish is tricky. This naturally healthy food is too often contaminated with unacceptable levels of neurotoxic mercury that is emitted from industrial facilities like coal plants, polluting the waterways in which fish live. It is especially dangerous to in-utero babies and children. Mercury accumulates as it goes up the food chain, which is why eating small fish like sardines and anchovies is much safer than eating larger fish like tuna. Then there's the issue of quality: Wild fish are typically higher in omega-3 fatty acids and are cleaner and safer, while most farmed fish are grown in overcrowded conditions where they're susceptible to parasites and infections, given antibiotics and hormones, and fed tainted, grain-based foods, and have a higher ratio of inflammatory omega-6 fatty acids to boot. But conversely, and confusingly, wild fishing is decimating fish supplies worldwide, while some new aquaculture (fish farm) operations *are* raising fish the right way. How to navigate this maze? Get educated. The Safina Center's Sustainable Seafood Program (safinacenter.org) and Seafood Watch (seafoodwatch.org) can help lay out the sustainability options of various fish, while EWG's Consumer Guide to Seafood has a calculator that evaluates mercury content and omega-3 levels, rates suggestions for your age and life stage, and tells you what kind of fish to choose and how much is safe.

TEA AND COFFEE

THE DRINKS THAT GET YOU THROUGH THE day also deserve scrutiny. Tea is a much greater carrier of pesticides than most people realize. Leaves are sprayed, not washed, and then infused directly into your boiling water. Plus many tea bags have plastics in them. Buy an organic brand like NuMi or Traditional Medicinals, or loose organic tea from Mountain Rose Herbs. Coffee is often grown in countries with few standards regulating chemicals, so the safest choice is to buy organic or from a small specialty roaster who deals directly with farmers and knows the story of their supply chain. (Small farmers and specialty roasters often don't have organic certification, but they may be using fully chemical-free processes and buying in smaller batches, decreasing the likelihood of toxic mold in the beans. Ask questions when you buy.) Also, decaffeinated coffee should be water-processed, not chemically processed, in order to reduce your exposure to unnecessary toxins.

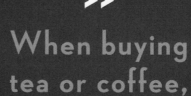

When buying
tea or coffee,
choose organic.

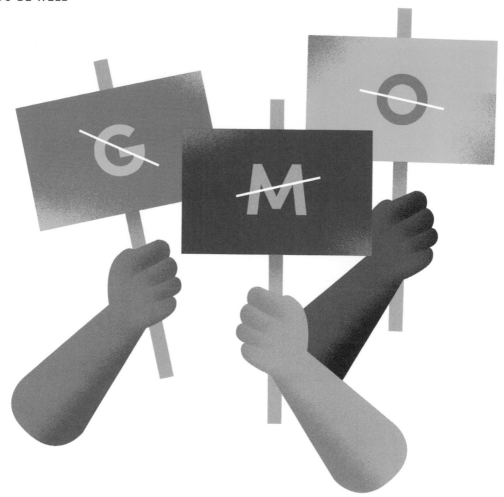

ADOPT THE PRECAUTIONARY PRINCIPLE: BOYCOTT GMOS

WHY DO MOST OF THE INTEGRATIVE-MEDICINE DOCTORS I KNOW SCRUPULOUSLY AVOID EATING FOODS MADE WITH GENETICALLY MODIFIED ORGANISMS (GMOS)? BECAUSE WE'VE SEEN SKYROCKETING CASES OF ASTHMA, ALLERGIES AND FOOD SENSITIVITIES, AUTOIMMUNE CONDITIONS, AND AUTISM IN THE TWO DECADES SINCE THESE

FOODS INFILTRATED OUR SUPPLY. CONVERSELY, WE have observed improvement of many of these conditions when GMOs and pesticide-laden foods are removed from the diet. We know enough to be extremely concerned, and though the correlations between GMOs and poor health aren't making headline news—often silenced by the dollar—we adopt the precautionary principle: *When evidence points toward potentially significant, widespread, or irreparable harm to health or the environment, options to avoid harm should be pursued, even if harm is not yet fully understood or proven.*

I believe strongly you should also follow this principle and refuse to be a guinea pig in this billion-dollar unmonitored and unregulated experiment. Instead, commit to eating organic food (which, by definition, is not genetically engineered) whenever you can, gradually lower your toxic load, and get to Know Your Sources (page 40) so you can make the best choices.

WHAT IS THE ISSUE?

A GMO (genetically modified organism) or GE (genetically engineered) food is created when the DNA of different species is fused to form a type of plant or food that does not exist in nature or is not created by traditional crossbreeding. Foreign genes from one species are extracted and artificially forced into the genes of an unrelated plant or animal, usually in a laboratory. This is primarily done to produce crops that can tolerate strong herbicides like Roundup (see page 153) or produce their own internal pesticides, theoretically to produce greater yield for less cost. The motivation is economic, not based on health or quality.

The main GE foods are soybeans and corn (and all their derivatives, from tofu and soybean oil to cornmeal, high-fructose corn syrup, and much more); cottonseed (fed to livestock and used in margarine); canola oil; sugar beets (and consequently, most "sugar" in processed foods that is not derived from pure cane sugar); and alfalfa (fed to livestock). The hormone given to dairy cows to increase milk supply (rBGH) is genetically engineered, as is the sweetener aspartame and some other food additives. It's estimated that 70 to 80 percent of processed foods in the U.S. contain GE ingredients. (GMO sweet corn, papaya, zucchini, and yellow summer squash are also for sale in grocery stores, but in far lesser amounts.) In case it's not obvious, GMO danger is one of the most persuasive reasons to steer clear of most processed and junk foods; do whatever you can to replace conventional animal products with certified organic, grass-fed, and most definitely rGBH-free; and, if you eat out frequently, think before you order in restaurants.

THE (VERY) RED FLAGS

Here are a few of the many reasons to be concerned about GMOs:

CONSUMING GMO FOODS has been linked to conditions such as neurological problems, reproductive issues, and gluten-related disorders.

THE BT TOXIN engineered into corn and cottonseed is a bacteria that makes the crops pest-resistant by creating tiny holes in insects' digestive tracts. Experts believe this could be to blame for the explosion in intestinal permeability in humans: When we eat these foods, and the meat, dairy, and eggs from animals that consume them, the toxin can create holes—or "leaky gut"—in us. This is a root cause of many diseases in modern times.

THE HERBICIDES used in tandem with GMO seeds have strong antibiotic properties and damage your gut flora.

THE RGBH HORMONE not only raises levels of IGF-1, a cancer-promoting hormone similar in structure to insulin, it also lowers the milk's nutritional status and creates increased antibiotic resistance in humans.

A GROWING MOUNTAIN OF SCIENTIFIC EVIDENCE from numerous feeding studies has demonstrated that GMOs have killed animals and sickened others by triggering reproductive problems and weakened immunity, and shortening life expectancies. (Note that residues of glyphosate allowed on animal feed can be 100 times that allowed on grains for human consumption.)

THE ECOLOGY OF AGRICULTURE IS CHANGING: Massively resistant "super weeds" are evolving and requiring conventional farmers to use more—and stronger—herbicides than ever before. It's a problem similar to antibiotic resistance in humans.

GMOS SPREAD EASILY to nearby non-GMO crops, and even organic crops, carried by wind. Contamination of the broader food supply is a very real problem.

To get up to speed on the most pressing issues around food safety, visit robynobrien.com, the website of health activist, and my good friend, **Robyn O'Brien**. Robyn has been called "food's Erin Brockovich," and she is not just an HTBW pro, she is one of my health heroes.

IT'S AN INSIDE JOB

GE foods, including the rGBH hormone, are highly restricted or banned in many nations, but the U.S. and Canada have approved them based on studies done by the very industry that produces and profits from them. Known as the biotech industry, it's largely based on the seed and pesticide companies Monsanto, Dow, Bayer, Syngenta, DuPont, and BASF, and with monopolistic mergers on the cards, don't expect a slowdown of GMO production anytime soon. Plus, the government officials who oversee this area are famously intertwined with the industries they regulate. Consumer demands for proper labeling, accountability, and transparency have been met with major pushback from the food industry and government agencies. But take heart: Market demand *does* change

the playing field. Notice how many dairy producers now tout their "rGBH-free" products and the plethora of brands bearing the non-GMO or GMO-free stamps. When you reject GE foods with your dollars, the food industry is forced to evolve.

WHAT TO DO ABOUT IT

To limit your exposure to GMO foods, follow the Institute for Responsible Technology's four-step protocol:

1.   BUY ORGANIC

2.   LOOK FOR NON-GMO PROJECT SEALS

3.   AVOID THE AT-RISK INGREDIENTS MENTIONED PREVIOUSLY

4.   BUY PRODUCTS LISTED IN THE NON-GMO SHOPPING GUIDE, available on the Institute for Responsible Technology website (responsibletechnology.org)

Also join the fight against GMOs by supporting the "Just Label It!" campaign (justlabelit.org) to change legislation so that GMO foods are clearly labeled, enabling consumers to make more informed purchasing choices.

When evidence points toward potentially significant, widespread, or irreparable harm to health or the environment, options to avoid harm should be pursued, even if harm is not yet fully understood or proven.

GLYPHOSATE: WOULD YOU LIKE SOME POISON ON THAT OATMEAL?

One of the most troubling aspects of GE food is the explosion of the use of Monsanto herbicide Roundup—the most widely used herbicide in the world. It is not only used during the cultivation of 80 percent of GE foods, but it's also sprayed on lots of non-GE crops to speed up harvesting. Conventional wheat, barley, rye, potatoes, sweet potatoes, edible beans, soy, corn, sugarcane, sunflower seed, buckwheat, millet, and more are all (according to organizations who report on biotech industry) routinely sprayed shortly before the crops are picked and then turned into your morning cereal or healthy vegetarian foodstuff! It's also widely sprayed in parks and gardens, along roads, and on golf courses—maybe even in your own apartment complex or your neighbors' yards.

The World Health Organization has classified the primary ingredient in this herbicide, glyphosate, as a probable carcinogen—an absolutely damning classification that the biotech industry fought tooth and nail to avoid—and countless stories of serious illness in farming communities are emerging. Studies show it kills the benevolent bacteria in your microbiome, and among the many side effects of ingesting it are reproductive problems; liver, kidney, and skin cell damage; and antibiotic resistance. It's shown to be an endocrine disruptor (even at the low levels permitted in tap water) and to kill beneficial gut bacteria. It also damages the DNA in human embryonic, placental, and umbilical cord cells and is linked to birth defects and reproductive problems in laboratory animals. Not surprisingly, one study showed chronically ill humans had higher glyphosate residues in their urine than healthy humans. Despite this, the EPA has for years failed to measure the levels of glyphosate on our foods like it does with other herbicides and pesticides (though this may now be changing due to consumer demand).

Unfortunately, because Roundup is the most widely used herbicide in the world, it pervades the entire food chain. It is in drinking water and even rainwater, in plants, animals, and the blood of every human tested so far! The devastating effects of glyphosate use will become a very big story in the next few years, but don't wait to clean up your diet (especially if you are already suffering from a chronic condition, planning to conceive a child, or have young children in your home). And be proactive about investigating whether herbicides are used by landscapers where you live and play.

Learn more about glyphosate at detoxproject.org, or read *Whitewash: The Story of a Weed Killer, Cancer, and the Corruption of Science*, by Carey Gillam, which exposes the corporate and government cover-ups behind this dangerous herbicide's explosive growth.

GET A WATER FILTER!

MAKE THIS SINGLE INVESTMENT IN YOUR HOME (AND WORKPLACE) INFRASTRUCTURE. IT IS NOT A SOFT-AND- FLUFFY LIFESTYLE CHOICE. IT'S A SAFETY MEASURE ON PAR WITH WEARING A SEATBELT OR LOOKING BOTH WAYS BEFORE CROSSING THE STREET. HERE'S WHY: TODAY'S TAP WATER IS EXPOSING YOU TO A COCKTAIL OF

UNWANTED CHEMICAL CONTAMINANTS. OF THE 316 chemical contaminants found by the Environmental Working Group in tap water nationwide, only 114 are subject to any government regulation or safety standards (and even these safety levels are unreliable, as they do not account for typical spikes in the supply). They include chlorine, fluorine compounds, disinfectant byproducts, pesticides, herbicides like glyphosate, and other volatile organic compounds, as well as assorted hormones from hormone medication and traces of other prescription drugs (which are especially problematic for pregnant women). They can even include highly fluorinated toxic chemicals from Teflon manufacturing known as PFCs, as well as traces of metals like arsenic and lead. Some of these things can hurt your liver, kidneys, and reproductive organs; many of them mess with your hormones; and others are linked to various medical conditions like obesity and cancer. The long-term effects of many of these contaminants, and their effects in combination with each other, are unknown.

TOXIN SPOTLIGHT: The chlorine used to treat water, while reducing bacteria that could cause water-borne diseases, does so at the cost of good bacteria in your gut. It also creates a huge array of disinfectant byproducts (including a dangerous group called trihalomethanes) that are suspected carcinogens and can be especially problematic for babies in utero. Most carbon filtration systems remove these byproducts.

A shower filter is just as important as a drinking-water filter, because your skin absorbs contaminants, too. In fact, ten minutes spent in the shower equates to drinking one gallon of water, and the chlorine byproducts are even more volatile in that hot, steamy environment. Shower filters are affordable and easy to install, and bath filters are

also available for your tub faucet. Aquasana and Berkey are just two of the brands making these.

WHAT KIND OF FILTER SHOULD I GET?

Any filter is better than none. While a whole-house filtration system is ideal, it is pricey. You'll probably want to start by looking for a drinking-water filter certified by the independent testing group NSF. To simplify, there are four major types:

UNDER THE SINK: Typically reverse osmosis filters, these remove the most contaminants, including the "rocket fuel" contaminant perchlorate, but they use a considerable amount of water to create each gallon of pure water.

COUNTERTOP: Carbon-block based, they remove more contaminants than pitcher systems.

FAUCET-MOUNTED: These remove most major contaminants, though may slow water flow slightly.

PITCHERS AND CARAFES: These remove considerable contaminants, but typically don't clear all the disinfectant byproducts or lead.

Whichever filtration system you use for drinking and bathing, change filters regularly, according to manufacturers' instructions, so it functions effectively.

Use the Environmental Working Group's Water Filter Buying Guide (at ewg.org) to get specific information on filter systems and what contaminants they remove. And start with their Tap Water Database to see how your municipal water stacks up.

PROTECT YOUR SKIN ECOLOGY

JUST AS YOUR GUT HAS AN ECOSYSTEM OF INFINITE BACTERIA THAT EXIST TO KEEP LIFE AND HEALTH IN BAL- ANCE, SO DOES YOUR SKIN. YOUR SKIN IS THE MAIN BARRIER BETWEEN YOUR INNER PHYSIOLOGY AND THE OUTSIDE WORLD, AND THE MICROBIOME NOT ONLY PROTECTS IT AGAINST PATHOGENS, IT ACTS AS ITS

IMMUNE SYSTEM. IT IS ALSO A MIRROR OF THE STATE of your inner health: When any of your systems, such as endocrine, digestive, or immune, are imbalanced, that may be reflected in the state of your skin. That's why tending to skin issues at the root causes rather than just topically—which for many people means eliminating aggravating foods (page 90) and repairing the gut (page 174)—is often a more effective means for clearing them up.

Also, just like with your gut, the microbiota (community of organisms) on your skin can experience a dysbiosis, which is an imbalance in which unhelpful bacteria take over and helpful bacteria get suppressed. When this occurs, you might experience skin irritation and disorders like acne, eczema, and rosacea, heightened sensitivity, slower healing, and more tendency to infection—or you just may not look quite as radiant as you'd like.

Take care of this all-important ecosystem by considering its needs every day. Antibacterials, high concentrations of drying alcohols, and harsh cleansing agents can upset the microbiome balance, strip the skin barrier (also called its "acid mantle") of its protective lipids, and disrupt its healthy pH level (which should be around 5.5). Products that are too alkaline (above a pH level of 9.0) or too acidic (below 3.0) should be avoided due to their potential to upset the biome and pH balance of healthy skin. Some forward-looking beauty companies address this directly. Drunk Elephant, a nontoxic brand developed to help restore the skin's natural, healthy state, lists the pH of its products on the box.

As research mounts about the importance of skin's microbiome and how to keep it healthy, beauty experts increasingly recommend that if you struggle with persistent skin issues, you should give your skin its own form of detox.

Often it's the stuff we *put on* our skin in an attempt to "fix" its issues that causes the problems. By removing the bad stuff—identifying and removing any alkaline, drying, or antibacterial formulas, and tempering the habit of cleansing in the morning, which can strip the acid mantle unnecessarily—imbalanced skin gets a "clean break," allowing its barrier and microbiome to recover on their own terms. Then you can feed and nourish the skin with good, clean ingredients in well-formulated products, just as you would nourish any other organ. A lifestyle that includes regular sweat sessions will support you on this quest: Perspiration from exercise, saunas, and especially outdoor activity (with a little dirt mixed in) is the ideal prescription for keeping your skin biome healthy because sweat supports the healthy balance of protective bacteria—it's like prebiotics for the probiotics on your skin!

There's another important reason to quit using antibacterial cleansing products on your face and body as well as in your home. The widespread adoption of these products correlates with a rise in allergies because they deprive us of natural immune-stimulating exposure to pathogens. Take sanitation too far and it can cause the much-needed diversity of flora in your microbiome to weaken.

Tip: If your day doesn't present options for a sweat-streaked blast of nature, you can spritz it on instead using ammonia-oxidizing bacteria facial sprays from companies like Mother Dirt. These deliver live probiotics to your skin to help restore its naturally balanced state.

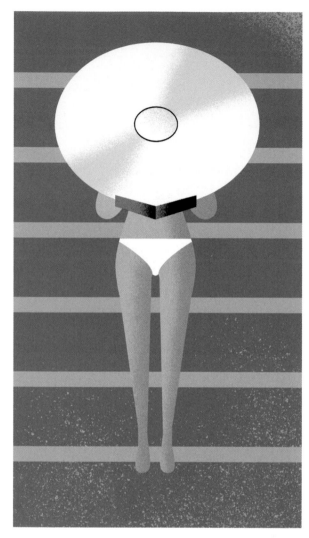

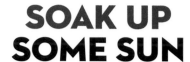

SOAK UP SOME SUN

WHAT IF YOU THOUGHT OF YOUR SKIN AS ONE BIG solar panel that converts waves of ultraviolet light into health-protecting vitamins and immunity-boosting energy? Your solar panel needs to be cared for thoughtfully and safely, of course, but it *wants* exposure to sunlight—something that is as essential to your functioning as food and water. Sunlight is the primary way your body makes vitamin D, a steroid with hormone-like activities, which regulates the function of over two hundred genes and is necessary for bone-building, inflammation control, neurological and cardiovascular function, fighting depression, and, very critically, preventing many kinds of cancer. (Food can provide some vitamin D, but in much lower amounts.) New science shows how sunlight also energizes the T cells that play a central role in your immunity. Yet indoorsy lifestyles have robbed us of this ultra-protective element: 80 percent of Americans are deficient in vitamin D, and we're only starting to understand what the consequences may be. I recommend testing your levels periodically if you can and, whenever possible, combining sensible sun exposure with supplementation as needed.

HOW TO GET YOUR D ON

In our all-or-nothing culture, we've lost a balanced relationship with the sun, either underestimating its power and burning or damaging our skin, or shirking it entirely. There is a middle road, however: developing a safe personal strategy for sun exposure.

First, it's important to understand that UVB rays are what help you generate vitamin D (though in excess, they also cause burning), while UVA rays contribute to aging and the damage that causes skin cancer. UVB rays only hit you when the sun is at an angle of 35 degrees above the horizon, so your body can only make vitamin D in the middle of the day, even in sunny places (but you can still

In our all-or-nothing culture, we've lost a balanced relationship with the sun.

suffer damage from UVA rays at any time). Your latitude and altitude also affect UVB rates: In winter, locations more than 35 degrees from the equator will not deliver UVB rays, so supplementation will be needed. One of the quickest ways to figure out how to get the best UVB exposure is to use an app called dminder, which, using your skin tone, age, body type, geographic location, and current weather, calculates how many minutes you need in the sun to generate optimal D without burning. (Note that UVA rays penetrate windows, but UVB rays do not. Don't try to sun yourself through glass.)

Now get outside! Daily exposure of large amounts of bare and unprotected skin to sunlight, for just the amount of time it takes before you become pink in any way, will optimize your D levels. This could be five minutes if you are very fair-skinned, or much more if you are dark-skinned and tend not to burn. Exposing yourself to sun in steady, incremental amounts will help you safely build to longer stints. The inexpensive SunFriend wristband can help you monitor your exposure and warn you when to cover up. Protect your face while in the sun, as this skin is delicate and prone to aging and wrinkles.

When you have reached your max for that day, cover up, seek shade, or use a healthy, chemical-free sunblock. A mineral-based product that uses zinc oxide or titanium to physically block sun rays by reflecting and scattering them is safest (it protects against both UVB and UVA rays). Also, don't overestimate the protection that sunblock gives. One of the primary causes of sunburn and skin cancer is the use of poor-quality sunscreens (which may prevent burning but don't properly defend against the UVA rays that cause melanoma) combined with a false sense of security: *If I've got sunblock on, I can stay out here for hours!* Reapply often, and be sensible about layering up with T-shirts, pants, hats, or rash guards if you are going to be outside for a long time.

Finally, but critically, stay boosted with supplementation as needed. When daily sunlight is not available, you will need a vitamin D_3 supplement. (D_3, aka cholecalciferol, is the type of vitamin D your body produces in response to sun exposure, while D_2, aka ergocalciferol, is a syn-

TEST YOUR VITAMIN D LEVELS

Reasonably priced testing kits from the Vitamin D Council offer an easy way to test yourself and your family. Testing twice a year in spring and fall is ideal. Most doctors look for an "adequate" reading of a serum 25(OH) D level greater than 20 ng/ml, but this number is on the low end. An optimal range of 50 to 80 ng/ml is where you want to be. (If your levels are low, it's wise to check with your doctor before leaping into excessive supplementation, especially if you are on medications such as cholesterol-lowering drugs, corticosteroids, and seizure medications, or have any kind of kidney disease.)

thetic form—avoid it.) Look for a D_3 supplement that is combined with vitamin K_2, and take it with a meal that includes some healthy fat because vitamin D is fat-soluble and requires some fat to be absorbed. Most people need anywhere between 2,000 and 10,000 units per day depending on their blood levels; higher doses should only be taken under doctor's supervision. Symptoms like a metallic taste in the mouth, increased thirst, itchy skin, muscle aches and pains, urinary frequency, nausea, and diarrhea and/or constipation can be signs that your D_3 dose may be too high, though this is rare.

BECOME A HEALTHIER HOUSEKEEPER

ENTIRE BOOKS ARE WRITTEN ON WAYS TO MINIMIZE THE TOXIC LOAD OF THE PRODUCTS AND FURNISHINGS YOU LIVE WITH. HERE'S WHY: THE EPA SAYS THAT POLLUTION INSIDE THE HOME CAN BE TWO TO FIVE TIMES GREATER THAN OUTSIDE, DUE TO IRRITANTS AND CONTAMINANTS IN THE PRODUCTS WE USE DAILY, OFF-GASSING

CHEMICALS FROM MATERIALS AND FURNISHINGS, AND even chlorine byproducts emitted from toilets (a good reason to keep the toilet lid closed). Household cleaners are not regulated by law or required to meet legal safety standards. Nor is it a requirement that their ingredients be listed, even though many of the most commonly used ones have been linked to asthma, cancer, reproductive disorders, hormone disruption, and neurotoxicity. From endocrine-disrupting phthalates in mystery "fragrances" to noxious fumes in oven cleaners, the impact and the synergistic reactions of multiple chemicals used together are largely unknown.

Unlike outdoor pollution, removing these interferences to being well is fairly easy to do. Start by using this stripped-down survival guide to mastering a greener and cleaner-for-you home.

REMOVE: THE MOST TOXIC CLEANING PRODUCTS

AIR FRESHENERS, EVEN THOSE LABELED "GREEN," "NATURAL," OR "WITH ESSENTIAL OILS." Studies that tested a range of air fresheners found they all emitted compounds classified as hazardous under U.S. federal laws, including carcinogenic ones. Instead, open windows, increase ventilation, and use fans, air purifiers, and essential oil diffusers.

ANTIBACTERIAL PRODUCTS FOR HANDS AND HOUSEHOLD. These contribute to drug-resistant bacteria.

FABRIC SOFTENERS AND DRYER SHEETS. Both have been shown to cause allergies or asthma and can irritate the lungs. Add a little vinegar in the rinse cycle instead.

DRAIN CLEANERS AND OVEN CLEANERS. These can burn eyes and skin. Instead, use a drain snake or plunger in drains, and try a DIY paste of baking soda and water in the oven.

REPLACE: CLEANERS WITH FAILING GRADES

When each bottle or pack of soap, detergent, spray, polish, or scrub runs out, take a minute to look at its rating on the Environmental Working Group's Guide to Healthy Cleaning. Be sure to rate your window cleaners (which may contain toxic solvents), harsh surface and toilet bowl cleaners, and anything fragranced, as fragrances typically use a cocktail of unknown ingredients including phthalates. If it's grade C or below—and especially if it has a warning of any kind on the packaging—use the guide to find a safer alternative. There are plenty on the market, and they can be easily ordered online if you can't find them in a store near you. Another option is DIY household cleaners made from baking soda, vinegar, and natural antibacterial and antifungal agents like tea tree oil, which are enjoying a resurgence and are extremely easy to make at very low cost (see page 160).

RETHINK: 4 HOUSEHOLD HEALTH HAZARDS

1. REPLACE PVC-CONTAINING SHOWER CURTAINS (which contain volatile organic compounds, phthalates, and metals, and are more volatile in a steamy environment)

with curtains made with natural alternatives like hemp or the stable and safer vinyl PEVA, or glass shower doors.

2. **SUBSTITUTE PARCHMENT PAPER OR BEESWAX CLOTH FOR PLASTIC FOOD WRAP,** which contains endocrine-disruptive compounds.

3. **INVEST IN A GOOD SET OF GLASS STORAGE CONTAINERS** and/or mason jars instead of using plastic food containers, because they also contain endocrine-disruptive compounds.

4. **RETIRE THE NONSTICK COOKWARE,** especially if it has been scratched. The perfluorinated chemicals used to make nonstick surfaces are extremely toxic, particularly when overheated. Try the ceramic-coated GreenPan for safer nonstick cooking.

REFRESH: YOUR CLEANING HABITS

If you dry-clean your clothes or curtains, find a cleaner that uses water-based technology (yes, this is okay despite "dry-clean only" labels) or liquid carbon dioxide, not neurotoxic chemical solvents like perchloroethylene. When hiring a carpet cleaner, ask similar questions about their process.

Invest in a high-quality, high-power vacuum that seals in dirt and dust to help minimize your exposure when emptying the collection chamber (look for one with a HEPA filter). Household dust and dirt is thought to be one of the biggest sources of exposure to endocrine disruptors. Take off your shoes when you come in from outside to minimize bringing in toxins like herbicides.

Always make sure the area you are cleaning is well ventilated.

RENOVATE WISELY

If you plan to undertake upgrades or renovations in your home, consider the implications of the materials that you live in, sit on, and sleep on. Organic mattresses, while an investment, pay back considerably when you consider that you lie on them for a third of your life. Safer, non-VOC paint costs only a little bit more than regular. (VOCs, or volatile organic compounds, are released into air as paint dries.) And be sure to investigate the toxicity of the flooring and carpeting you are considering and look into alternatives like sustainable surfaces or wool carpeting (which tends to be free of chemical treatments). When replacing old carpeting, take care to remove it quickly and aerate the room because it may contain phased-out fire retardants that off-gas from underneath.

Household cleaners are not regulated by law or required to meet legal safety standards.

10 BAKING SODA CLEANING HACKS FROM ANNIE B. BOND, GREEN LIVING EXPERT

A commonly available mineral full of many cleaning attributes, baking soda is made from soda ash and is slightly alkaline (its pH is around 8.1; 7 is neutral). It neutralizes acid-based odors in water and absorbs odors from the air.

1. **DRAIN CLEANER:** Pour 1 cup of baking soda down the drain, followed by 3 cups of boiling water.

2. **CHEMICAL SMELLS FROM CLOTHES:** Mix 1 cup of baking soda into a tub of water and soak clothes for two to three hours or overnight. Agitate occasionally. Repeat if necessary, and wash as usual. (This method is great for removing the new smell from clothes.)

3. **CAT URINE ON RUGS AND FABRIC:** Alternate sprinkling on baking soda, which will neutralize acid odors, with white distilled vinegar.

4. **DOG ODORS AND URINE ON RUGS AND FABRIC:** Sprinkle with baking soda. Let set for a few hours before sweeping up.

5. **SILVER POLISH:** Make a paste from ½ cup baking soda and a few tablespoons of water. Scoop some onto a clean, soft rag and rub onto the silver. Rinse with water and polish dry.

7. **SOFT SCRUBBER:** Pour about ½ cup of baking soda into a bowl and add enough liquid soap or detergent to make a frosting-like texture. Scoop onto a sponge and use to clean your bathtub or tiles. Rinse with water.

8. **SCOURING POWDER:** Simply sprinkle baking soda into a sink or tub and scrub.

9. **OVEN CLEANER:** Sprinkle baking soda onto the bottom of the oven. Squirt with enough water to dampen. Let set overnight, making sure the baking soda is still damp before you go to bed. In the morning, simply scoop the baking soda and grime out with a sponge and rinse.

10. **REFRIGERATOR DEODORIZER:** Place an open box in the back of the fridge. It will absorb odors by drawing them to the baking soda molecules.

11. **CUTTING BOARD DEODORIZER:** Sprinkle the cutting board with baking soda, scrub, and rinse.

Be as aware of what you put ON your body as what you put IN your body.

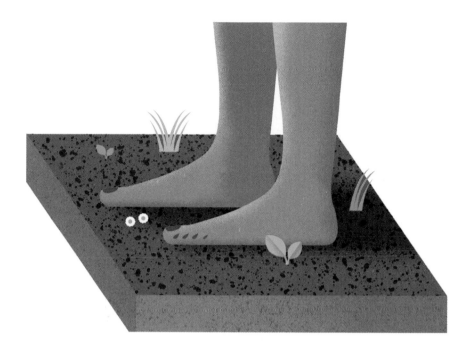

LOSE THE SHOES!

IF YOU'VE EVER FELT BETTER AFTER A BAREFOOT WALK ON THE BEACH, OR SLEPT BETTER ON A WILD-AND-
FREE VACATION IN NATURE, AN EMERGING BODY OF SCIENCE CALLED EARTHING IS EXPLAINING WHY: WHEN YOU TAKE OFF YOUR SHOES AND WALK ON THE EARTH, OR SIMPLY SIT OR LIE ON THE GRASS, YOU ARE HARNESSING

THE NATURAL NEGATIVE ELECTRICAL CHARGE OF THE earth. This replenishes your supply of free antioxidant electrons, which helps to stabilize your body's bioelectrical systems, promote anti-inflammatory activity by neutralizing positively charged free radicals, and regulate your biorhythms. In an impressive array of studies, this practice, colloquially called "earthing," reduced every measure of stress tested. Perhaps no surprise, it's also been shown to be an effective way to restore orderly rhythms of wake and sleep because it helps resynchronize cortisol to its proper patterns.

I'm not sure we even need science to point us in the right direction here because it's common sense: When you feel the ground under your naked feet, you begin to relax, you breathe better, and your nervous system settles down. You feel rejuvenated afterward—perhaps a little clearer in your thinking, too. Sand, dirt, grass, gravel, and, to a lesser extent, even concrete are conducive surfaces for this most humble of health-promoting acts. So kick off your shoes; stand, sit, or play in the grass; take your lunch to the park; and use your movement breaks (page 126) to get outside. (And if you want to improve morale in the office, get your colleagues involved in a game of barefoot soccer, tag, or bocce!) A daily dose of contact with the earth can help buffer the tsunami of stress that is a part of everyday existence and make you more resilient and energized—try it for a week and see.

GREEN THE WAY YOU GROOM AND PAMPER

WHAT IF THE CRITERION YOU USED TO EVALUATE YOUR SKINCARE PRODUCTS WERE THAT YOU COULD ONLY APPLY THEM IF YOU COULD SAFELY EAT THEM, TOO? GIVEN THE EXTREMELY LARGE SURFACE AREA OF THE SKIN (IT'S YOUR LARGEST ORGAN), ITS HIGHLY PERMEABLE AND POROUS NATURE, AND ITS EXTREME SENSITIVITY

TO TOXIC CHEMICALS, THIS ISN'T SUCH A WILD DE-mand, as what we put on our skin enters and then affects our bodies as much (or maybe even more than) what we ingest! However, I'd advise you not to try that in today's world: Over the past two decades, the European Union has banned more than 1,300 chemicals used in personal care products and restricted the levels of over 250 more. To date, the United States has only partially banned thirty.

HOW TO BE WELL EXPERT **Gregg Renfrew,** a longtime patient and friend, is the founder of Beautycounter, a brand that is changing the face of clean beauty. This is how she suggests tackling the project of minimizing unintentional exposure to toxins in self-care products:

Start with products that cover the largest part of your body, like body wash, body lotion, sunblock, and so on. Use the Never List from beautycounter.com for guidance; it lists the over 1,500 questionable or harmful ingredients we prohibit in our formulations, including the top worst offenders like parabens, phthalates, and fragrance, and you can download a wallet-sized version of it to reference while shopping. If any ingredient on the list is in a product you're considering, you know to steer clear of it. Additionally, the Environmental Working Group's Healthy Living app, which includes their famous Skin Deep guide to safe self-care products, is a great resource to use while shopping to see how your products rank.

What many people don't know about personal-care products is that terms like "natural," "botanical," and "organic" have no meaning in the beauty industry, so doing your own research matters. And while you might assume that "natural" cosmetics are inherently safer, in fact, heavy metals like lead and cadmium are naturally occurring and often contaminate natural cosmetics. When seeking safer products, know that not all natural brands are safe and not all synthetic colorants are unsafe. My simple tip is to look for beauty brands that screen their color cosmetics, preferably each batch, for heavy metals.

It's also important to realize that your voice matters. I've seen firsthand how individuals can have a significant impact in transforming the beauty industry. You can join the growing movement for cleaner cosmetics by asking our elected leaders for new laws on the beauty industry. To take action, simply text "BetterBeauty" to 52886 to receive a link whereby you can email your representatives.

Another guide to help as you shop is the Think Dirty app from thinkdirtyapp.com.

WHICH TO SWITCH

Focus on switching out products you apply most often and leave on the longest, or that make contact with the most intimate and permeable tissues in your body. When you run out of a product, seek a safer, nontoxic alternative, and within a few months you will have stocked a cleaner collection.

SKIN LOTION: It's applied all over the body and left on to absorb deeply. Lotions are frequently made with parabens and petrochemicals.

SUNSCREEN: Look for mineral-based sunblock to reduce exposure to carcinogenic compounds in conventional sunscreen.

DEODORANT: Applied under the arms near the lymph nodes, which are close to your breast tissue and where absorption is extremely high. Conventional deodorant typically contains aluminum, a metal of concern linked to neurological and other problems.

HAIR RELAXERS AND COLORANTS (ESPECIALLY THOSE MARKETED TO AFRICAN AMERICAN WOMEN): These are some of the most toxic products out there. Be sure to rate yours using the Skin Deep guide.

FEMININE HYGIENE PRODUCTS: Choose organic cotton or consider a menstrual cup. Conventional cotton in these intimate products may be bleached with carcinogenic chemicals and contain traces of glyphosate.

LUBRICANTS: Standard lubricants can contain petroleum and parabens. Look for authentic toxin-free products, like those from Sustain Natural.

SCRUBS, WASHES, AND TOOTHPASTES WITH MICROBEADS: Microbeads are damaging to aquatic life after they enter waterways, and then they return, toxin-filled, in your drinking water.

MOUTHWASHES: The alcohol dries out the mouth, increasing the risk for oral cancer. Try the traditional art of oil pulling to naturally increase oral hygiene.

ANYTHING ANTIBACTERIAL: The active ingredient triclosan is linked to thyroid disruption and liver and inhalation toxicity, and it harms aquatic life after entering waterways. It's still found in some toothpastes and other personal care products.

PRODUCTS CONTAINING "FRAGRANCE": Under international intellectual property law, the word "fragrance" can have many harmful ingredients hidden behind it and companies don't have to list them on the label.

THE LEXICON OF PERSONAL-CARE INGREdients can make your mind melt, so here's a quick cheat to use as you shop: If the first few ingredients listed contain sodium lauryl (or laureth) sulfate or petrochemicals like propylene glycol, paraffin, mineral oil, butylene glycol, isopropyl alcohol, and/or petrolatum, or if the bottom ingredients contain fragrance (or parfum), DEA (diethanolamine), MEA (monoethanolamine), TEA (triethanolamine), and/or any parabens (butylparaben, propylparaben, methylparaben, and ethylparaben), it's a sign to put the product down and look for something cleaner.

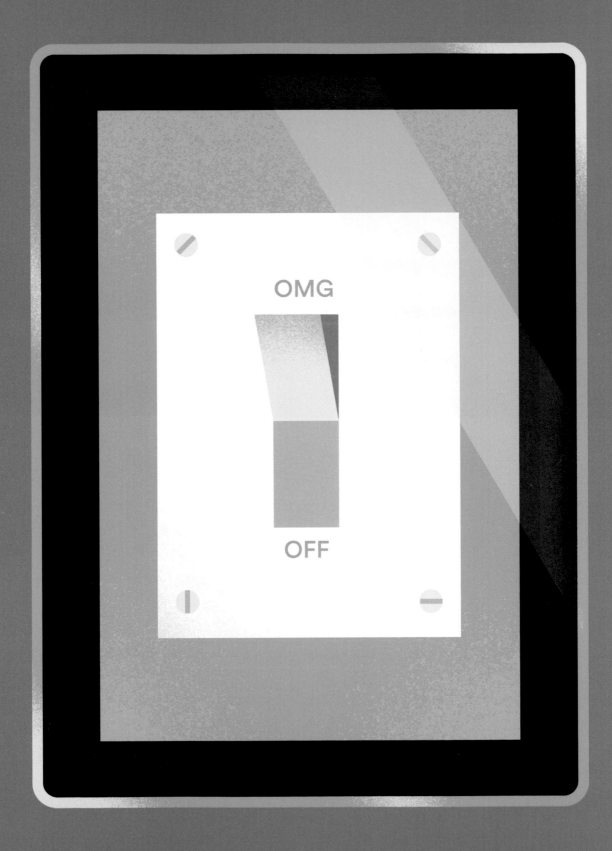

OMG EMFS!

IF YOU'RE CONSTANTLY TIRED, IRRITABLE, UNABLE TO FOCUS AT WORK OR HOME, OR HAVING HEADACHES OR INSOMNIA, TURN OFF YOUR ROUTER AND POWER DOWN THE CELL PHONE. FOR THAT MATTER, IF YOU'RE HEALTHY AND WANT TO *STAY* HEALTHY, TURN OFF YOUR ROUTER AND POWER DOWN THE CELL PHONE, AT LEAST AT

NIGHT, WHEN STUDIES HAVE SHOWN THAT THE BODY is most vulnerable to their stressful electromagnetic frequencies (and when your body very much needs to rest and repair).

For the average person, the biological effects of the electromagnetic energy emitted by communication technologies—as well as from things like the electrical wiring in your walls—are impossible to see and difficult to measure. But these invisible forces—frequencies of energy like light, but man-made, not natural—are interacting with your biology all day and night, and medicine is just starting to understand the dysregulating impact.

For the last several decades, reams of scientific literature have been alerting us to how radiation from cell phones, communications towers, Wi-Fi routers, smart meters, and antennas present a system-wide, biologically disruptive phenomenon. This phenomenon not only impacts our ability to function well, sleep, and think clearly, it also causes damage at the cellular and molecular level, which can lead to cancer (and impact the blood-brain barrier, cardiovascular system, immune system, stress response, and much more). In 2011, The World Health Organization's International Agency for Research on Cancer (IARC) classified this band of radiation, which is known as radio-frequency radiation, as Group 2B "Possible Carcinogen," and there are calls based on more recent science to upgrade this. Esteemed scientists around the globe say this is a growing environmental health crisis and one that we are largely asleep to. In the U.S., the wireless industry is now preparing to install ultra-high-frequency 5G antennae—what is sometimes called "Wi-Fi on steroids" and is literally military-grade technology—on utility poles throughout neighborhoods, mere feet from people's homes, possibly with no local oversight or intervention if they get their way.

It's relatively easy to talk about the behavioral problems like compulsion and distraction associated with technology (page 186), but the conversation about the invisible *biological* effects makes everyone uncomfortable because it is all around us and feels so out of our control. Yet as we stand at the dawn of the "internet of things"—in which homes are filled with smart technologies, cars drive themselves, and your watch is constantly beaming information gathered from your body—concerned experts are saying that our mitochondria, which evolved to respond to only *natural* types of electromagnetic frequency (like sunlight and electrons from the Earth's surface), are becoming stressed beyond their capacity and there exists the need for society to rethink its relationship with technology. We must appreciate the ways in which wireless technologies interfere with the electrical systems in our bodies, and choose technologies that minimize these exposures. This becomes even more important as we add more and more technology to our living environments.

Clinicians are starting to see the connection between wireless radiation exposure and the extraordinary growth in chronic illnesses, which includes seeing illnesses in children that previously were only seen in elderly patients. Anecdotally, many patients and doctors alike have reported that chronic symptoms like headaches, behavioral issues, or insomnia have receded through small EMF-reducing interventions, which can have a big impact. Wireless reduction strategies are especially important if you have children in your family, because their bodies and brains are still developing; they are also important for the elderly, where symptoms from wireless radiation exposures can be mistaken for the signs of aging.

We can't afford to live in denial. Use the following guidelines to reduce your exposure to EMFs, and stay abreast of new developments through watchdog and educational sites like manhattanneighbors.org and ehtrust.org. Your health, and that of your family, may depend on it.

PRACTICE GOOD CELL HYGIENE. Never hold your phone to your head to talk. Instead, use it in speaker-phone mode or with an air tube headset; text instead of calling whenever possible; and try not to use it when signal quality is poor. Don't wear it on your body while it's switched on. Whenever possible, use a hard-wired corded phone (cordless phones emit high radiation), or use Skype or Facetime on your hard-wired computer to make calls. Reduce your cell use in cars, even with head-sets—the radiation gets magnified when it reflects off metal. Don't use a cell phone near pregnant women and young children, and never let a child use a cell phone—the radiation permeates their skulls much more powerfully.

CLEAN UP YOUR TECH HABITS. Never work with your laptop on your lap, and if you have a wireless rout-er, turn it off at night; to be extra safe, switch your inter-net connection back to a wired Ethernet cable instead of wireless. When you're not online, turn off your comput-er or device's wireless connectivity software (including Bluetooth and AirPort). Switch to wired external key-boards, mouses, and printers (printers are a very high source of exposure). And learn the risks of smart meters installed on your home and the ways to mitigate them at takebackyourpower.net, or check out emfsafetystore.com for their Smart Meter Shield Kit and other shielding and EMF measurement supplies. You can also have a "Building Biology" specialist assess your exposure levels to EMFs, as well as other toxins like mold, in your home or office and advise on health-supporting changes. (Find a Build-ing Biology specialist at hbelc.org.)

GET WISE AND GET INVOLVED. Stay informed and do your part with citizens groups like ElectromagneticHealth. org, the Environmental Health Trust, and the EMF Safe-ty Network.

We must appreciate the ways in which wireless technologies interfere with the electrical systems in our bodies.

THINK ABOUT YOUR DRINK

MY PERSONAL POINT OF VIEW IS THAT ALCOHOL IS a toxin that harms the liver, kills brain cells, alters the microbiome, and disrupts sleep, and that when it comes to some beers, ciders, liquors, and liqueurs, it's also a significant source of carbs that could otherwise be avoided. (Most of my patients who drink wine daily, even dry wine, tend to put on weight and store fat.) But I'm well aware that I'm in the minority here, and the millions of city dwellers I live among definitely don't agree! Drinking is a part of life for many people, and a way to connect and commune. If that's the case for you, I simply invite you to gently consider how and why you drink, to determine if it's a habit done automatically or a pleasurable ritual that fills you with well-being. There are four questions that are worth asking yourself in order to understand your relationship to alcohol:

IS THAT GLASS OF WINE, beer, or cocktail a treat you truly relish, sip by sip, or a default drink you pour each night, without much consideration?

IS YOUR DRINK OF CHOICE an enriching enhancement to your meal or social experience, or is it your way of medicating stress, anxiety, or a lack of joy, or helping you lose inhibitions that otherwise hold you back?

DO YOU TEND TO DRINK ALONE, or with a partner or in a group setting—and in each case, why?

ARE YOU HAPPY WITH YOUR relationship to alcohol, or is there something you'd like to change about it?

Context is everything when it comes to drinking. Tuning in to why you're drinking and being conscious of its purpose each time you do it is a powerful tool for keeping your relationship with alcohol in healthy balance. Check out the resources at betterdrinkingculture.org.

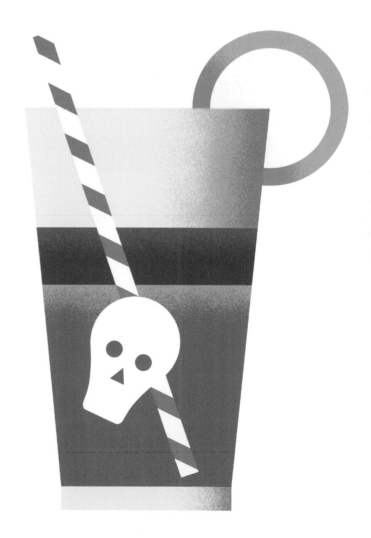

GIVE YOUR MITOCHONDRIA WHAT THEY NEED

YOUR MITOCHONDRIA ARE YOUR ENERGY POWERHOUSES: THE TINY FACTORIES IN YOUR CELLS THAT TURN THE FOOD YOU EAT AND OXYGEN YOU BREATHE INTO ENERGY IN THE FORM OF ATP, OR ADENOSINE TRIPHOSPHATE, WHICH POWERS THE BIOCHEMICAL REACTIONS IN YOUR CELLS. THEY ARE ESPECIALLY ABUNDANT

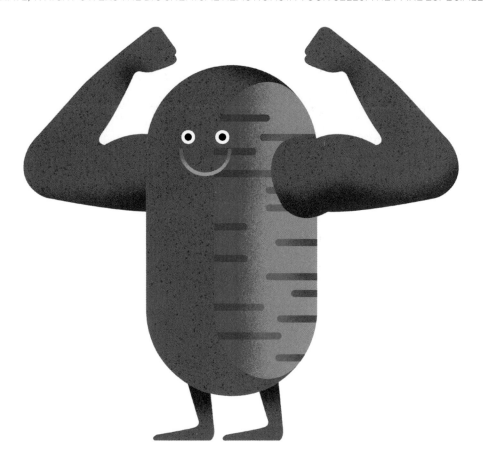

IN THE CELLS OF YOUR HEART, BRAIN, AND MUSCLES, which demand the most energy. Though you likely don't think about them, the vitality of your mitochondria is pivotal to how energetic you feel, how robust your metabolism is, and how clearly you think. And like a factory that slows down production when resources run low or con- ditions are poor, mitochondria produce less energy when they don't get the raw materials they need; encounter too much stress; are exposed to toxins, electromagnetic frequencies, infections, or allergens; or are trying to do their work in an overly sedentary body.

You will start hearing about mitochondria more and more as science is finding long-anticipated answers to the mysteries about how they work. I believe that your mitochondria are likely the mechanism by which lifestyle changes like diet, exercise, sleep, and sunbathing initiate meaningful improvements in how you function and feel—I also see mitochondria as the Western equivalent of *chi*, the essential force of life and longevity that is so deliberately cared for and protected in traditional Chinese medicine.

Mitochondrial deterioration is at the root of the fatigue we associate with getting older and is possibly related to heart disease, lung disease, neurodegenerative diseases, and age-related diseases, but you can do something to fix that. The more you boost your mitochondrial function and quantity, the better you will feel and the more gracefully you will age.

>>

The more you boost your mitochondrial function and quantity, the better you will feel and the more gracefully you will age.

<<

Initiate fourteen essential habits to slow the deterioration of your mitochondria.

1. QUIT EATING SUGAR. Mitochondria don't like using sugar as food.

2. ADOPT A GRAIN-FREE DIET to further limit the amount of sugar in your blood.

3. EAT MORE VEGETABLES to gain more nourishing phytonutrients.

4. CONSUME PLENTY OF HEALTHY FATS. These are the preferred fuel of mitochondria.

5. EAT CLEAN. Pesticides and toxins damage mitochondria.

6. PRACTICE INTERMITTENT FASTING.

7. DEVELOP A ROUTINE OF HIGH-INTENSITY INTERVAL TRAINING. HIIT has been shown to make more mitochondria.

8. GET STRONG. There is more mitochondria in lean muscle mass than in fat.

9. PRACTICE BETTER SLEEP HYGIENE.

10. SOAK UP SOME SUN. Sunlight is a powerful mitochondrial booster.

11. AVOID ELECTROMAGNETIC RADIATION.

12. START YOUR DAY WITH A COLD SHOWER. Cold exposure, in short bursts, helps trigger the production of new mitochondria.

13. TAKE SUPPLEMENTS. CoQ10, glutathione, magnesium, B vitamins, krill oil, alpha-lipoic acid, nicotinamide riboside, and PQQ (pyrroloquinoline quinone) are key sources of mitochondrial support.

14. REDUCE EXTRANEOUS MEDICATIONS. A number of medications, including statin drugs, antidepressants, and antianxiety medications, have been documented to reduce mitochondrial function.

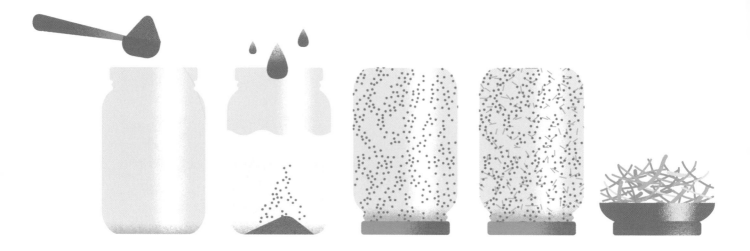

GROW YOUR OWN SPROUTS

TURN A CORNER OF YOUR KITCHEN COUNTER INTO A MINI VEGETABLE GARDEN. SPROUTS ARE A VEGETABLE POWER FOOD: VERY INEXPENSIVE, A CINCH TO GROW, AND PACKED WITH ENZYMES THAT HELP YOUR BODY EXTRACT NUTRITION (THINK: VITAMINS, MINERALS, AMINO ACIDS, AND ESSENTIAL FATS) FROM OTHER FOODS.

SPROUTS ARE THE JUST-POPPING GROWTH OF A PLANT seed—the first iteration of a new plant. All it takes to sprout is a few basic supplies, a very small dose of TLC (two minutes a day for three to five days), and bingo, you have a supply of supercharged plant food to add a boost to your meals. A sprout habit pays back not only with fresh veggies but also prodigious detoxifying and protective benefits. Broccoli sprouts in particular are known for their extremely high levels of cancer-fighting compounds, especially one called sulforaphane that kickstarts the release of the liver's detoxification enzymes. Soaking and sprouting is a game-changing technique that you can also use to reduce the inflammatory lectin content of beans, legumes, and grains.

PICK YOUR SEEDS. You can sprout a spectrum of plant foods! There are leafy sprouts, brassica sprouts, bean sprouts, and more. Start with a universally pleasing and easy-to-source brassica like mildly peppery arugula or broccoli, and always look for "sprouting" seeds from a good organic/non-GMO source. Then, once you've got broccoli and its brethren growing, explore other types of seeds to expand your repertoire.

GET SPROUTING. All you need is a quart-sized canning jar and a widemouthed canning ring plus a mesh sprouting screen (or a plastic "sprouting lid"). Alternatively, an Easy Sprout Sprouter can be purchased for less than $15.

GROW YOUR OWN SPROUTS

STEP 1   At night, pour about 3 tablespoons of sprouting seeds into your canning jar. Place the sprouting screen over the top of the jar and screw on the canning ring. Pour about 2 cups of non-chlorinated water through the screen. To increase the mineral content, add a piece of kombu (a type of seaweed) to the jar before adding the water. Swirl the seeds, drain, and then cover again with about 2 cups of water. Leave the jar on your counter overnight.

STEP 2   In the morning, drain the water and remove the kombu if used. Add another 2 cups water and then rinse, swirl, and drain again. Once drained, lay the jar on its side at a slight angle (prop it up using a bowl with a rim, or a pan with something that wedges the bottom of the jar up an inch or two).

STEP 3   Two to three times per day, drain the old water, rinse with fresh water, and drain again. The seeds should be moist but free of standing water. (If you see furry white "cilia" clouds on the sprout tails, they need a little more moisture in the jar—add a few drops and shake gently.) Place the jar back on its side. Watch your sprouts sprout! They should start to fill the jar, gradually turning green. This takes three to five days, and sometimes longer for greens.

STEP 4   When the sprouts look quite long and green, shake them into a bowl, wrap them gently in a paper towel, and store in a plastic bag in the fridge. Keeping your sprouts dry helps stop growth and limits spoilage.

STEP 5   Enjoy a handful of sprouts per day on salads and soups or even blended into smoothies! Use within five days.

Sproutpeople.com is an excellent source for quality sprouting-seed supplies.

All it takes to sprout is a few basic supplies, a very small dose of TLC, and bingo, you have a supply of supercharged plant food to add a boost to your meals.

CREATE A SMART
SUPPLEMENT STRATEGY

IN A PERFECT WORLD, NO ONE WOULD NEED SUPPLEMENTS. OUR FOOD WOULD CONTRIBUTE THE OPTIMAL NUTRITION TO FUND EVERY BIOCHEMICAL ACTION OF THE BODY EASILY AND FLAWLESSLY AND KEEP US ENERGIZED AND RESILIENT AS WE AGE. GIVEN THAT IT'S *NOT* A PERFECT WORLD AND THAT THE NUTRITIONAL

QUALITY OF FOOD (EVEN HEALTHFULLY GROWN AND produced food) has degraded while stressors of all kinds have increased, I consider high-quality supplements to be essential health boosters. They're not substitutes for a good diet, but they can help fill the gaps left by a compromised food system, replenish the nutrients that are burned up by exposure to chemicals (the body uses more nutrients to protect you) and in times of stress or little sleep, and aid with the inevitable decrease in nutritional absorption as you age. Supplements are important because if the raw materials required for metabolic reactions aren't coming from food, the body will scavenge them from your bones, liver, or other tissues, which takes a toll on your energy and health.

THE STRATEGY WHEN IT COMES TO SUPPLEMENTATION SHOULD BE:

1. ALWAYS FOCUS ON EATING THE BEST DIET YOU CAN first and foremost.

2. BUY THE BEST-QUALITY SUPPLEMENTS YOU CAN AFFORD; one or two good ones outweigh multiple poor-quality ones.

3. IF GOOD-QUALITY SUPPLEMENTS ARE COST PROHIBITIVE, focus on high-quality food, exercise, sleep, and stress reduction instead.

While there are many excellent supplements that you can use to build a program of support targeted to your needs, there are a few I recommend as a baseline protocol:

A GOOD MULTIVITAMIN that contains vitamin D, B vitamins, and magnesium. Multivitamin supplements play a crucial part in all metabolic process of the body, including assisting in energy generation and promoting growth, reproduction, and health of cells. A good multivitamin is the foundation of health and nutrition. Avoid the one-a-day kind—they can never contain the amount of minerals you need. Do look for ones containing methylated forms of vitamin B_{12} (methylcobalamin) and folic acid (as L-5-methyltetrahydrofolate) because many people have minor genetic defects that interfere with optimal methylation, a process central to detoxification, inflammation control, immune function, and more. Take your multi with food to enhance its absorption. If you are on any medications, review your multivitamin's ingredients with your doctor to ensure there are no contraindications. *Note: In sunless months, most people will need extra vitamin D supplementation in addition to a multivitamin. Aim for a combined total amount of at least 2,000 IUs a day unless blood tests indicate greater need. (For more information on vitamin D, see page 156.)*

HIGH-QUALITY FISH OIL. Fish oils contain the omega-3s that support your body's ability to prevent chronic diseases and help protect it against inflammation. They also keep skin, hair, and nails healthy, enhance your focus, and stabilize your mood. My preference is krill oil over other types of fish oil (krill are small, shrimp-like crustaceans that feed on phytoplankton) because it also contains astaxanthin, a powerful antioxidant. Given the high levels of contamination in fish, krill is a safe and low-toxic way to get your supply of essential fatty acids because it is so low on the food chain and harvested in clean waters. Of all the sources of omega-3s, krill oil is the most environmentally sustainable. Make sure it is cold-processed, not processed with chemical solvents, and when buying any fish oil, choose a brand that has been tested for mercury.

A PROBIOTIC. If you are consuming a diverse array of fermented foods throughout the week (see page 54), you can get away without a probiotic, but if not, include one daily—at least 20 billion CFUs for everyday use, double that if you're prescribed antibiotics—rotating brands every couple of months to ensure you get diverse strains. (If you are taking, or have recently finished, a course of antibiotics, be sure to take the probiotic at a different time of day than when you take the antibiotic, and include the strain *Saccharomyces boulardii*.)

Two additional supplements that can deliver extra support, particularly as you get older, are GLUTATHIONE and COQ10, which are made in the body but decrease with age. These antiaging antioxidants improve mitochondrial function—and your energy levels. Look for acetylated glutathione for maximum absorption, and ubiquinol CoQ10 for the same reason.

It's important to buy supplements that use the best ingredients and are free of harmful preservatives, fillers, binders, excipients, anticaking agents, shellacs, coloring agents, gluten, yeast, and lactose and other allergens. The "top tier" brands, available from health practitioners, include my line Be Well, Thorne Research, Ortho Molecular Products, Designs for Health, Metagenics, Xymogen, LifeExtension, and Pure Encapsulations. The next tier down, a little less potent but still safe and available at health-food stores, includes Jarrow Formulas, Garden of Life, Bluebonnet, KAL, Source Naturals, Solaray, and Renew Life. The website labdoor.com evaluates supplements for safety, efficiency, and purity—its database is still small, but it can provide useful snapshots on mainstream brands.

Supplements are important, because if the raw materials required for metabolic reactions aren't coming from food, the body will scavenge them from your bones, liver, or other tissues.

REPAIR YOUR GUT

TWO OF THE MOST IMPORTANT THINGS YOU CAN DO FOR YOUR HEALTH ARE PROTECT YOUR GUT MICROBIOME AND REVERSE ANY GUT DYSFUNCTION THAT IS OCCURRING. IN SIMPLEST TERMS, AN IMBALANCED MICROBIOME OCCURS WHEN THE PRO-INFLAMMATORY SPECIES OF BACTERIA IN THE GUT DOMINATE THE ANTI-INFLAMMATORY

SPECIES, AND WHEN THE PROPER DIVERSITY OF SPEcies in the gut is highly compromised. This is caused by many of the factors described throughout this book, including highly processed and genetically engineered foods, chemical inputs and medications, hyper hygiene, chronic stress, poor sleep, and lack of exercise. Unfortunately, an imbalanced microbiome is a fairly common state of affairs, and it goes hand-in-hand with leaky gut: Over time, the inflammatory toxins released by the imbalance, along with damaging effects from the stressors mentioned above, combine to make the gut wall's one-cell-thick lining lose its integrity. The cells' tight junctions start to weaken and let partially undigested food particles and toxins slip through, into the bloodstream. This triggers inflammation and a slew of immune-system hyper reactions. When you consider that this gut wall lining has the total surface area of a tennis court but is thinner than tissue paper, you can imagine how influential it is to your whole physiology— and how easy it is to damage!

The symptoms that result from leaky gut can extend far beyond expected digestive problems like gas or bloating, or even obvious food sensitivities and allergies. They can present as anxiety and depression, brain fog and mood swings, skin problems (like acne and rosacea), joint pain, muscle aches, fatigue, weight issues, and a weak immune system, plus more serious problems like autoimmune diseases, asthma, and, according to new research, possibly even diabetes and obesity.

The good news is that you can rebalance your microbiome and help repair the gut wall lining through diet, supplements, and stress reduction—no drugs necessary (in fact, some pharmaceutical drugs prescribed to manage inflammation due to leaky gut will make things worse). The microbiome is a flexible, living ecosystem that changes constantly, and the cells in the intestinal lining replace themselves every three to six days. As a result, with some commitment on your part, you can personally oversee a resilient rebuilding project that has the potential to turn your health around.

One of the best ways to execute this repair program is to use a formula called the 5Rs. The 5Rs give you a basic template from which to create your own month-long repair protocol based on homemade food; it also forms the basis of well-designed detoxifying programs that use medical-grade nutrition and supplements (such as my Be Well cleanse). I've given you an overview of the 5Rs; for more detailed guidelines on creating your own 5R program or to discover ready-made programs that support this repair work, visit howtobewell.com.

>> **An out-of-balance microbiome can present with anxiety, depression, brain fog, sleep issues, and even memory problems.** <<

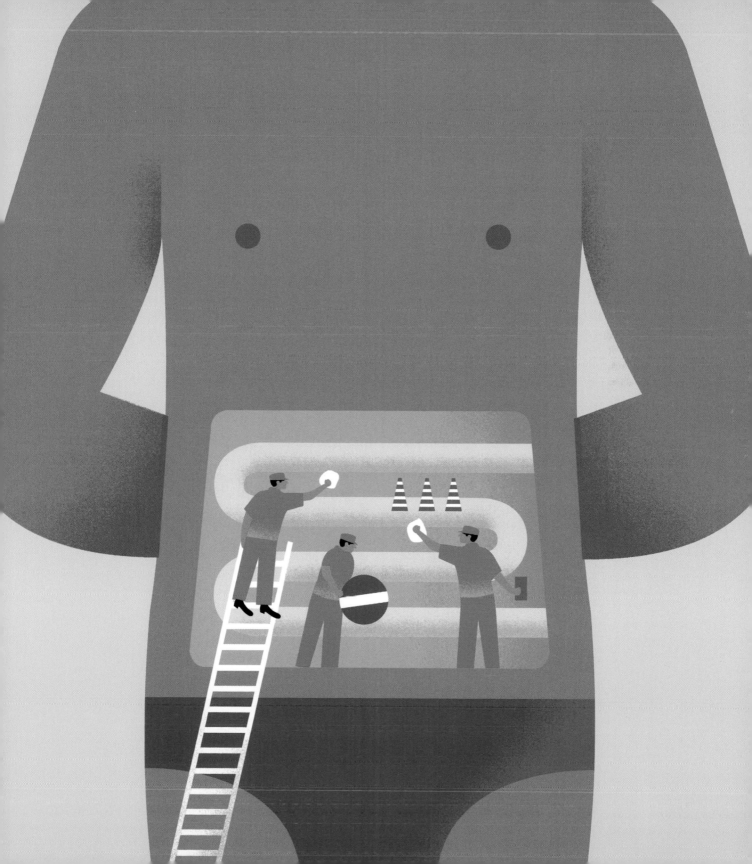

REMOVE THE SOURCES OF IRRITATION

DIETARY TOXINS: These include sugar and processed foods, factory-farmed animal products, pesticide-laden foods, artificial sweeteners, and GMOs.

FOODS THAT TRIGGER SENSITIVITIES: You can determine this by using an elimination diet (page 90).

GASTRIC IRRITANTS: Such as alcohol and caffeine. With your doctor's supervision, limit or try to completely do away with nonsteroidal anti-inflammatory drugs and proton pump inhibitors.

CHRONIC LOW-GRADE INFECTIONS: Small intestinal bacterial overgrowth (SIBO), yeast/candida overgrowth, and parasites living in the intestines are extremely common. A knowledgeable healthcare provider can help diagnose and treat these with herbal antimicrobials (and occasionally medications if necessary).

REPLACE WHAT MAY BE LACKING

FIBER helps eliminate toxins and byproducts of food through the large intestine. Without fiber, your bowels move slowly, allowing waste to reenter the system and create inflammation and toxicity throughout your body. Eat an array of colorful nonstarchy vegetables, berries, nuts, seeds, and some legumes, and/or supplement with 1 to 2 tablespoons of psyllium seeds, flaxseeds (grind these yourself in a clean coffee or spice grinder to ensure freshness), or soaked chia seeds.

HYDROCHLORIC ACID is required to start the digestive process. If it is depleted, natural "bitters" before meals can help stimulate gastric juices, as can a tablespoon of apple cider vinegar mixed in some water. A supplement of hydrochloric acid is sometimes required and is best introduced under a health professional's supervision.

DIGESTIVE ENZYMES help to break down food and make nutrients easier to absorb and assimilate. The more food is broken down, the fewer problems come from partially digested and potentially irritating food particles.

REINOCULATE WITH BENEFICIAL BACTERIA TO REESTABLISH A HEALTHY BALANCE OF MICROFLORA

DAILY PROBIOTICS support and rejuvenate the microbiome to rebalance, assist with digestion, help your body make vitamins, aid in the absorption of minerals, strengthen the immune system, improve metabolism, and affect your mood.

FERMENTED FOODS (page 54) support this even further.

PREBIOTIC FOODS (page 57) act as fertilizer for the good bacteria.

PHAGES are the new story in gut supplementation, and some of the latest probiotic blends include them. Short for "bacteriophages," these are beneficial viruses that infect and kill microbes, help the beneficial bacteria to reproduce, and even protect the epithelial layer in the gut by concentrating in the mucus layer that protects that lining.

REPAIR THE GUT LINING WITH THE GOOD BUILDING BLOCKS IT NEEDS

GLUTAMINE SUPPLEMENTS support immunity and digestion by fueling the cells that line the small intestine.

OMEGA-3 FATTY ACIDS from a well-sourced supplement (page 172) help the gut rebuild healthy cell walls and improve the tight junctions between the gut lining's cells.

A GOOD MULTIVITAMIN (page 172) helps to remedy the nutrient deficiencies that commonly accompany leaky gut syndrome, even in those eating a healthy whole-food diet.

BONE BROTH (page 43) is full of gut-healing and soothing nutrients like collagen and gelatin.

A DIVERSE WHOLE-FOODS DIET replete with non-starchy vegetables, healthy proteins, and good fats delivers the vitamins, minerals, fatty acids, amino acids, and phytonutrients needed to repair damage and rebuild healthy new tissue, plus the enzymes the small intestine needs to heal. Include a diverse array of health-building foods to encourage a robust microbiome that can act as your reliable blockade against infection and disease.

RELAX TO KEEP STRESS AT BAY AND ENCOURAGE BETTER SLEEP

MINDFULNESS and other stress-reduction techniques support your healthier gut, as stress can lead to bacterial overgrowth, leaky gut, and inflammation.

. . . and don't forget to EAT MINDFULLY (page 66)!

Two of the most important things you can do for your health are protect your gut microbiome and reverse any gut dysfunction that is occurring.

BOOST YOUR DETOX FUNCTIONS

TWO TYPES OF TOXINS ADD UP TO CREATE THE TOTAL BURDEN ON YOUR BODY: ENDOGENOUS, WHICH ARE CREATED AS NATURAL WASTE PRODUCTS OF METABOLIC PROCESSES, AND EXOGENOUS, WHICH INCLUDE ENVIRONMENTAL INPUTS SUCH AS CHEMICALS AND HEAVY METALS. TO SUPPORT YOUR BODY'S ABILITY TO DETOXIFY ITSELF OF BOTH, TRY THESE TWO SIMPLE HABITS:

SWEAT

Work up a good sweat regularly. It helps flush out toxins from the body and control body temperature. Intense exercise and hot yoga are two ways to do this; saunas, especially infrared, are another. Saunas and similar heat treatments have been part of preventive health protocols for eons: their heat stimulates circulation, which lowers blood pressure, relaxes tight muscles, eases minor aches and pains, helps balance cortisol, and is shown to improve the functioning of the arteries by supporting the endothelial cells that line them. When you're feeling sick, saunas also help by boosting the immune system's white blood cell response to invaders, making them especially protective. Infrared saunas are my preferred option because they run at a lower heat than conventional ones, making them safer for those who can't tolerate high heat. The infrared waves penetrate deeply despite that lower temperature, helping to generate more profuse sweating that excretes more toxins. Aim for a couple of relaxing fifteen- to twenty-minute saunas per week, and be sure to stay well hydrated and shower right after so as not to reabsorb toxins. (You can find infrared saunas at gyms, yoga studios, and dedicated locations near you, or consider installing your own from companies like Clearlight and Sunlighten.

BRUSH

Dry brushing your skin before bathing helps it regenerate. Your skin is your largest organ, and it is responsible for 10 to 15 percent of body elimination. By gently sloughing away the dead cells that are left as skin regenerates, you decrease the load on the major detoxification organs: the kidney and liver. Dry brushing also aids in blood circulation and has a profound cleansing effect on the lymphatic system, an important filtration system that helps push toxins through and out of your body. It only takes three to five minutes to do this small self-care act. Here's how:

Purchase a natural fiber body brush from a health-food store or online natural lifestyle retailer—long-handled ones are best, for those harder-to-reach areas

STEP 1 Starting at your hands, run the brush up each arm toward the heart several times, covering all areas.

STEP 2 Stroke the brush from your feet to the tops of your legs in the same way.

STEP 3 Use circular clockwise strokes on your abdomen and armpits. Then repeat these areas with a counter-clockwise motion.

STEP 4 Brush your chest/breasts and any sensitive areas of skin lightly.

STEP 5 Brush upward over your back and then down from your neck. You can also brush in a circular motion on the palms of your hands and soles of your feet.

STEP 6 You can end with a warm shower or bath, followed by a toxin-free body oil or lotion. Then relax and enjoy the benefits!

>>

"People are fed by the food industry, which pays no attention to health, and are treated by the health industry, which pays no attention to food."
—Wendell Berry

<<

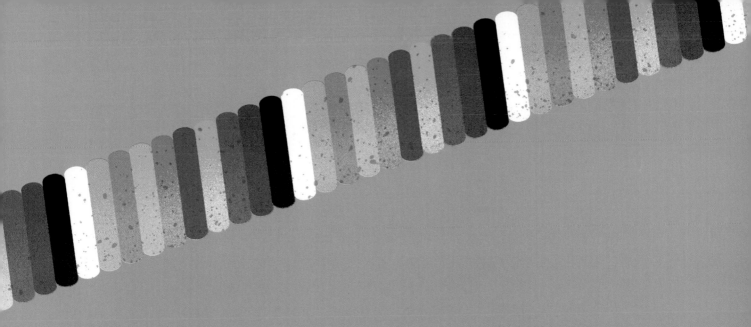

UNWIND

HOW DID WE LOSE SIGHT OF THE "OFF" BUTTON—AND at what cost? Most of us live in a state of almost permanent "on," by necessity if not by choice. The demands of work, family, relationships, and debts, plus the pressures to perform, produce, and perfect ourselves have never been higher (or existed so simultaneously, at every age and stage of life). The powerful "attention economy" of technology and media forces conspires to keep us online and hooked in to endlessly updating streams of information. It can be mind-bogglingly challenging to find points of stillness and relief: moments to unwind the hyped-up mind and relax the tensed body, to come back to your center, find clarity, and touch peace.

But finding these moments is a must. When you are subjected to ongoing mental and physical demands but deprived of rest and recovery, your whole nervous system takes a toll. You have heightened stress responses, which not only feel terrible, they negatively impact every system in your body, create anxiety, and disrupt sleep. You can lose resolve around food and movement—when stress creeps in, good habits can creep out. And you can get tangled in negative thinking that sabotages your best efforts to be well.

Unwinding is central to healthcare in many wellness traditions. Meditation, mindfulness, breath work, and soothing touch are not luxurious extras, they are daily essentials for managing imbalance and maintaining the body's healing power. You may not be able to escape to an exotic spa or Zen retreat—or magic away all the stressors you face—but these things aren't a prerequisite to unwind. Just invite some low-intensity into every day. Carve out small moments to relax, restore, and just "be." And know that these quieter habits are not pampering or self-indulgent. Just as night follows day and winter follows summer, stillness must follow activity—they are two sides of one whole.

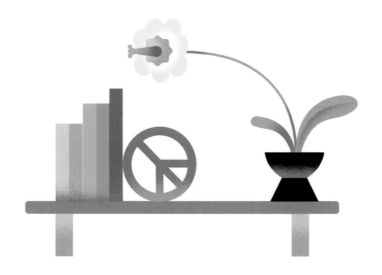

CLEAR YOUR SPACE,
CLEAR YOUR MIND

ARE THERE MOUNTAINS OF LAUNDRY IN YOUR BEDROOM, DIRTY DISHES IN YOUR SINK, PILES OF PAPERS TAKING OVER YOUR DESK? WHEN WAS THE LAST TIME YOU CLEANED OUT YOUR CLOSET OR GARAGE OR REORGANIZED YOUR OFFICE? IF YOUR HOME OR WORKPLACE IS CLUTTERED AND CHAOTIC, THERE'S A GOOD

CHANCE THAT YOUR HEAD IS, TOO. I'M REMINDED OF the quote that goes something like "the state of your space represents the state of your mind." Organization experts believe that space and mind work seamlessly together, so it's tough to know which came first, the clutter or the overwhelm. What *is* clear, however, is that a disorganized space can make you feel even more disorganized by supporting negative thoughts that zap you of hope and motivation. Every time you glance at that growing peak of laundry/dishes/papers, it's easy to think, *I'll never get my life together. I'm always behind. Everyone else is doing better than me.* Then, before you know it, these thoughts have become the guiding principles of your life.

Unlike other aspects of existence that really *are* bigger than you, you have complete control over the state of your space: You are the one who decides if you can't find your bed because it's covered in unfolded laundry. Yes, life is full, and it's easy to deprioritize cleanliness and organization, but small daily efforts—and creative

organizing hacks—can help you maintain your spaces so you can focus on the things that really matter. A good start is to adopt a philosophy of never putting off doing something that takes five minutes or less to do. Emptying the dishwasher? Five minutes. Folding the laundry? About five minutes. Putting your clothes away? Five minutes.

You can also limit clutter by making it easy to keep things off the floor or from piling up in common spaces. Containers are key. **Kim Colwell**, interior designer, feng shui expert, and friend of Be Well, suggests placing decorative baskets in each room of the house to give you and your family attractive, practical receptacles to house unfolded laundry, toys, or newspapers and magazines. You can buy inexpensive baskets at Ikea or garage sales (keep your eye out for these treasures) and spray-paint them interesting colors. You can also drape attractive fabric over the tops so you don't have to see their contents until you have the time to attend to them.

HOW TO BE WELL EXPERT

YOUR BREATH AS A
PATHWAY TO PEACE AND CALM

YOUR BREATH IS THE MOST EFFECTIVE, ALL-NATURAL EMOTIONAL MANAGEMENT TOOL THAT YOU'RE PROBABLY NOT TAKING ADVANTAGE OF. FREE AND EVER-AVAILABLE, BREATHING IS A SUREFIRE ROUTE TO CALMING THE MIND AND RELAXING THE BODY, YET MOST OF US TAKE IT FOR GRANTED. LIKE BLINKING, BREATHING IS A BODILY

FUNCTION THAT IS BOTH INVOLUNTARY AND VOLuntary. You breathe all day every day, rarely noticing the air entering and exiting your lungs, but this action takes on new power and meaning when you use it intentionally.

Bring your attention to your breath and you'll begin to make connections between how you feel and the way you're breathing. There is a clear link between your emotional state and your breath: When you're afraid you hold it; when you're anxious or stressed, it's quick and shallow; and when you're relaxed and happy, your breathing is slow and deep. This all happens unconsciously, as a natural reaction to outside stimuli or the content of your thoughts. On the flip side, you have the ability to use your breath to regulate your emotions. Deliberately breathing deeply, in and out, in a slow and steady fashion, reduces the heart rate and activates the calming part of the nervous system. This is why we instinctively ask someone who is visibly upset to "take a deep breath." Conscious breathing disrupts the swirling vortex of anxiety that's become a fixture of our go-go-go culture; it slows emotional reactivity and gives us access to our intuition, helping us make better decisions. When your breath is deep and steady, you are grounded, clear, and focused.

You don't need to be a meditation guru or yoga practitioner to tap into the power of the breath. Conscious breathing is easy to learn and can be practiced anywhere at any time: at your desk, sitting in traffic, or on line at the post office. I recommend that clients start slowly, by spending a few days simply bringing their attention to their breathing, an act that mostly goes unnoticed. Check in with your breathing right now: Is it speedy and shallow, located primarily in your chest and throat, or are your breaths longer and deeper, coming from your diaphragm and belly? From there you can experiment with altering your breathing patterns, extending the inhalations and exhalations, feeling your lungs and ribcage expand as you draw in air, and contract as you expel it. As you become more familiar with your breath and more confident in your ability to breathe consciously (instead of being "breathed" unconsciously), there are a few simple and powerful exercises you can practice whenever you'd like to feel less anxious and more grounded, or simply want to relax deeply.

You don't need to be a meditation guru or yoga practitioner to tap into the power of the breath.

BELLY BREATHING 101

Place your hands on your belly just below your lowest ribs. With your mouth closed, bring the tip of your tongue behind your top front teeth where they meet your gums. Take a slow, deep inhalation through your nose. Draw your breath all the way into your belly instead of breathing shallowly into the chest. Notice your diaphragm moving downward and, with your hands, feel your belly and ribcage filling like an expanding balloon. When you can take in no more air, exhale slowly through your nose until all the air is out of your lungs—you'll feel your belly falling under your hands. Breathe this way for ten rounds (a complete inhalation and exhalation is one round). As you continue, see if you can extend the exhalation, aiming for an out breath that is twice as long as the in breath. Breathing this way will help to quiet spinning and anxious thinking, and bring you back into your body and the present moment.

THE 4-7-8 BREATH

Your breath is an ally that can support you through emotional turbulence. The next time you find yourself swept away by anger, fear, anxiety, or extreme sadness, activate your built-in calming system. I recommend the 4-7-8 breath for an easy and effective way to soothe your nervous system and find your center again. You can use this technique whenever you're struggling emotionally or when you need to prepare for a performance of any kind.

To start, place the tip of your tongue behind your top front teeth at the gum line. Purse your lips as if you are going to blow out a candle and exhale completely through your mouth, making a whooshing or sighing sound. Then close your mouth and inhale through your nose for four counts, hold the breath for seven counts, and exhale back through the mouth for eight counts. Repeat this breathing cycle for ten rounds.

WHILE THE BELLY BREATHING AND 4-7-8 techniques come from long lineages of pranayama or yogic breathing, the vanguard of intentional breathing is a method devised by an iconoclastic Dutch adventurer named Wim Hof. His technique involves a series of deep, rhythmic inhales and exhales, followed by moments of holding the breath. Proponents—which include many high-performing athletes and plenty of ordinary people, including members of my Be Well team—say they feel energized, clear-minded, and focused as well as stronger and more physically capable after the practice, which in its fullest expression involves an invigorating (but optional!) cold shower. Credible research has shown immune system benefits—as well as inflammation and pain-reduction benefits—from the technique, which markedly increases oxygen saturation in cells and helps the body perform more effectively (and the optional cold shower appears to help ramp up fat metabolism and boost mitochondrial function, page 168). If you are curious about using the breath to maximize performance, go to wimhofmethod.com, and note that it's important to follow all the cautions listed on the website—this is not a practice for pregnant women, those with cardiovascular or other serious conditions, or those intending to take a bath or go swimming right after.

TAME THE **TECH BEAST**

WE LIVE IN AN ERA OF INFINITE SCROLLING AND ENDLESS CONNECTIVITY. OUR DEVICES ARE OUR CONSTANT COMPANIONS, STASHED IN OUR POCKETS THROUGHOUT THE DAY AND—ALL TOO OFTEN—BY OUR BEDSIDE ALL NIGHT. JAMMED WITH APPS TO HELP US TRAVEL, EAT, SHOP, AND EVEN MOVE MORE EFFICIENTLY, OUR

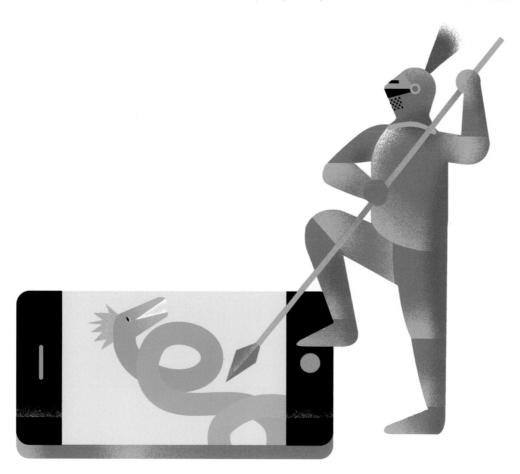

SMARTPHONES ARE CLOSE TO OUTSMARTING US. THE statistics are staggering: The average American child between eight and eighteen is in front of a screen for seven hours each day. Seventy-four percent of teenagers check their devices every hour, and most teens send about 3,400 texts a month. Their parents aren't much better—the average adult checks her phone every 13 minutes.

While the benefits of technology are real and plentiful—increased productivity, access to vast amounts of information, support in achieving and maintaining our goals—we are now experiencing the harmful side effects of our near-ceaseless techno-binging. At the top of the list is hyperconnectivity. Gone is the time when workdays had finite beginnings and endings. It's now possible, sometimes even expected, to bring your work to the dinner table and your kids' soccer matches, all at the expense of necessary downtime, real-life connections with family and friends, and your natural biorhythms. And it's become a norm to live in a cascade of interruption, as notifications ping us and push information into our mental space, hijacking our attention.

Nonstop access to social media, news feeds, and constant streams of information dissolves the boundaries that keep us balanced and healthy. Being incessantly clicked-in disrupts our ability to make and maintain genuine human connections, get deep and adequate sleep each night, and feel content with our own lives. We feel obligated to keep up, to show up, and to check in, voraciously consuming photos and videos of the perfectly curated lives of others instead of living fully in our own realities.

The more we gaze longingly at our colleague's dreamy-looking Caribbean vacation, the more we feed a cycle of unmet desires powered by a super-savvy algorithm. My in-house psychiatrist, Dr. Ellen Vora, calls this the "evil genius" of social media. When you hover over shots of someone's exotic getaway or a particularly intoxicating pair of shoes, you'll start to see *more* vacations and *more* shoes in your feed, perpetuating the belief that everyone is more well traveled (and well shod) than you. "There is a real 'echo chamber' effect that can reinforce whatever hypothesis you have about how the world works. It's all fake news in a way," Ellen says. "You can get really swept up and draw conclusions. Meanwhile, you are not enriching your inner life, say, with good literature, or relating to people, or exploring the world. We are effectively marketed to by corporations that exist to make you feel you must purchase, strive, and improve at all times. We are not encouraged to do the things that make us love the ones that we live with and be content with what we have."

There are a few disturbing clues that can tell you if you've been sucked into the vortex of a technology addiction. Have you ever strategically planned to have an actual interaction with an actual human being, requesting a face-to-face meeting with a quickly typed "IRL" (in real life), a text acronym that feels straight out of *The Twilight Zone*? Or maybe you have to consciously include "analog" experiences in your life, such as a picnic in the park or dinner for two. These real-life experiences are becoming the exception, not the norm. It's not entirely your fault: Checking Instagram for likes, Facebook for updates, and inboxes for the next email or text activates the same

The average American child between eight and eighteen is in front of a screen for seven hours each day.

pleasure receptors in the brain as drugs and alcohol. You get a rush of the happy hormone dopamine, but the search for the next high takes a toll, from tech injuries (page 128) and dry eyes (sometimes you even forget to blink!) to anxiety brought on by FOMO (fear of missing out), comparing yourself to others, and depressing news feeds. The biochemical impact of constant exposure to the electromagnetic fields (page 165) and blue light emitted from our electronics (page 102) adds further layers of invisible disruption.

The flood of products and content designed to keep you hooked in is not going to cease anytime soon. Creating an alternative digital reality in which *you* set the boundaries can be daunting but it's definitely within reach, and it can quite drastically improve your state of mind and quality of life. I recommend there be at least one room in your house, or one period during the day, where it looks like you're in the 1950s, free from a pixilated screen of any kind. This is the "tech-free" zone, and all family members and visitors must adhere to its rules. Then pick a few of the easy-to-implement tactics from the following list to help wrestle your life back from technology (while still remaining connected in the places that you need to be).

10 SMART TACTICS OF DIGITAL SELF DEFENSE

1. MAKE THE COMMITMENT TO PUT YOUR PHONE AWAY DURING MEALS you share with others.

2. TAKE A WEEKLY TECHNOLOGY FAST by dedicating one full day (Saturday or Sunday works well) to keeping your devices tucked away. Consider it a digital Sabbath.

3. CREATE TECH-FREE PERIODS during car rides or commuting. Dedicate these times to conversation, games, music, meditation, rest, reading, or quiet.

4. TURN OFF ALL NOTIFICATIONS (for new emails and messages) for every application on your computer as well as your phone and portable devices.

5. CREATE AUTOMATIC MESSAGES for your time away from devices to let people know that you check messages only during specific time slots. This will alert them that your response times may be delayed.

6. USE TECHNOLOGY TO MANAGE YOUR TECH HABIT. Apps like Moment, Freedom, and BreakFree place timers on internet and social media use—or even block them entirely for chunks of time—so you can build a healthier, more balanced relationship with your devices.

7. MAKE THE MAIN SCREEN ON YOUR PHONE HOME TO *ONLY* THE VERY BASIC APPS for phone calls, texting, and maps. This will reduce the temptation to engage. Hide time-sucking apps like Facebook in folders on the second or third page to make them harder to access.

8. SAVE ARTICLES YOU WANT TO READ using the Pocket app rather than wasting time when you don't have it on "must-read" stories, and install an app called Intently, which replaces advertisements with inspirational quotes and images on your browser.

9. TAKE THE BOLD STANCE OF REMOVING YOURSELF FROM ALL SOCIAL MEDIA and see what happens. Notice how you feel about not tracking the daily comings and goings of your friends and followers, and how much more time you have to do other things.

10. CONSIDER LEAVING YOUR PHONE AT HOME! Remind yourself that the likelihood of an emergency that necessitates you be reachable is fairly low, and meanwhile, you'll remember what it's like to initiate your own communication and have deeper conversation.

If technology addiction is taking over your family, I recommend the books *Glow Kids: How Screen Addiction is Hijacking Our Kids—and How to Break the Trance* by Nicholas Kardaras, PhD, and *The Hacking of the American Mind* by Robert Lustig, MD.

EMBRACE
OPTIMISM

WHEN TIMES ARE HARD AND YOU'RE FEELING
insecure, unsure, or simply unhappy, it's natural to feel
the pull to share your feelings with others. Yet continually
voicing your difficulties can push you down a rabbit hole
of negativity, ironically leading to increased disconnection
from others, a poorer outlook on life, and even compromised
health. Optimism may seem like an inauthentic approach,
but choosing to see the good in life is just that—a choice.
Actively directing yourself toward a sunnier outlook doesn't
have to be forced, and you don't have to jump from rain
clouds to rainbows in a day. Instead, make a commitment
to navigate the everyday happenings of your life from a
slightly brighter perspective. This can be as easy as noticing
your tendency to complain about things like the weather,
your boss, your significant other, or your kids and cutting it
off at the pass. Do this by focusing on the good that's also
in that situation or relationship. The good is always there.

THE WORLD'S SIMPLEST
OPTIMISM EXERCISE

Before you brush your teeth each morning, pause. Take ten
seconds to look at yourself in the mirror, breathe calmly,
become present to yourself, and commit to seeing the good
throughout your day. (A sticky note on the mirror might
remind you to do this daily.) Whether you call it gratitude,
appreciation, or thankfulness, become accountable to
yourself by deciding to appreciate what you have instead
of lamenting what seems to be lacking. Commitment
made, brush your teeth! Then, before you fall asleep at
night, take thirty seconds to review your optimism habit:
How did you do today? Did the complaints outweigh the
appreciation? Simply take notice, then let it go. Tomorrow
is another day.

>>

**Optimism is
learnable.
Just like eating
well or staying
fit, it becomes
easier with a
little practice.**

<<

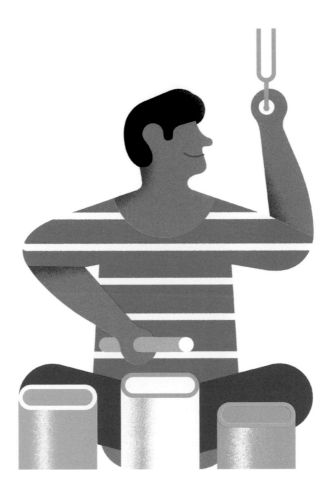

LISTEN UP!
THE HEALING POWER OF SOUND

CHANCES ARE STRONG THAT MUSIC IS ALREADY AN ESTABLISHED PART OF YOUR LIFE. OUR SOUNDTRACKS FOLLOW US, PUMPING THROUGH OUR HEADPHONES AS WE COMMUTE TO WORK AND HIT THE GYM, AND THROUGH OUR SPEAKERS IN THE CAR AND AT HOME. WHETHER YOU KNOW IT OR NOT, YOU USE MUSIC TO

ENERGIZE, MOTIVATE, COMFORT, AND SOOTHE. HOW often have you caught yourself humming a tune, singing an addictively poppy chorus, or tapping your foot to an irresistible beat? We all do it! Music is part of the human condition, as ancient and primal as we are, and it's good for us, too. Research continues to prove that music has

the capacity to be so much more than a pleasant addition to a given moment.

I often include music in healing protocols for my patients, strategically playing calming tunes during acupuncture sessions. The right music can induce an alpha state in a human being, that relaxed but alert feeling you find yourself in when activity ceases and you get a moment to reflect and recharge. When your brain is in alpha mode, you are liberated from the vise grip of never-ending to-do lists, nonstop social media updates, the 24-hour (bad) news cycle, and all of the anxiety they can produce. It's like a spa vacation for your nervous system, a state that can be consciously evoked and something that should be a required recharge for all twenty-first-century beings. Sound healing can even induce a theta state—one step beyond alpha, the slow-frequency brain state you get when drifting off to sleep or immersed in free-floating daydreams. Accessing alpha and theta states are not only about relaxation, though; research has found that they are when the body does some of its most profound healing.

Dropping into an alpha or theta state requires the right type of music. While techno or heavy metal may speak to you, they're not invited to this party. The music must have fewer beats per minute than your resting heart rate to guide you into space of calm and healing. Choosing music in the sixty BPM range is usually a safe bet, though you can also check out tracks composed of binaural beats (page 111). The work of Jonathan Goldman is often my first choice for helping my patients access those quieter states of body and mind. Jonathan is a premier sound healer, an expert in the field of harmonics, and his music is downright otherworldly, weaving together sounds from ancient religions, harmonics, mantras, and multicultural musical traditions. This is not the canned new age music of the past.

I encourage everyone to enjoy multiple doses of musical medicine.

4 WAYS TO HEAL WITH SOUND

1. DOWNLOAD ONE OF JONATHAN GOLDMAN'S ALBUMS onto your phone (I recommend *Frequencies*, for a "best-of" overview of his sound-healing repertoire) for relaxation and healing anytime, anywhere, though it's best to avoid operating heavy machinery (including your car!) after you press play.

2. ATTEND A SOUND BATH. This emerging wellness phenomenon marries deep, intentional relaxation with sonic-wave healing. Some yoga classes now feature live music like cello, harmonium, or flute, with or without vocalists. You can also search for local "sound meditations" and "sound baths" at wellness studios, spas, acupuncture clinics, and festivals—even some boutique hotels!—in which you lie in a state of relaxation while practitioners create relaxing, stress-busting soundscapes using kundalini yoga gongs, crystal bowls, tuning forks, or synthesizers tuned to specific frequencies. (A side benefit: Sound bathers report that slipping into theta state, the bandwidth of intuition and insight, stimulates greater self-awareness and creativity.) There are even hybrid experiences fusing meditation, music, and hands-on modalities, or small doses of cannabis-derived CBD oils for extra-relaxing effect.

3. If those sound too dreamy for you, PARTICIPATE IN A DRUM CIRCLE OR DRUM HEALING SESSION. Drumming in a group, using hand drums, is deployed to treat stress or trauma, enliven tired nervous systems, and quell anxiety and depression—and basically connect you to your primal self and empower you from the inside out. Plus, it's incredibly fun.

4. LISTEN TO NATURE SOUNDS like ocean swells and bird songs. Whether at home or at work, this is another restorative option that creates an infectious state of calm in you and those who enter your space.

MINDFULNESS:
AN ESSENTIAL TOOL IN THE MODERN HUMAN'S TOOLBOX

"MINDFULNESS" IS A KEY WORD OF THE CONTEMPORARY SELF-AWARENESS MOVEMENT, A LOFTY-SOUNDING TERM THAT INVOKES SOMETHING VAGUELY SPIRITUAL, BUT I SEE IT AS MUCH SIMPLER THAN THAT. IN MY OWN LIFE, AND FOR MY PATIENTS, I FRAME MINDFULNESS AS THE ANTIDOTE TO THE MULTITASKING EPIDEMIC

PLAGUING MUCH OF MODERN EXISTENCE. HOW OFTEN do you talk on the phone while driving? Fold laundry while watching TV? Interact with your kids while making dinner? Check Facebook while standing on line at the supermarket? Doing multiple things at once may seem like a normal, even practical approach to managing a busy life, but this relentless juggling of tasks is taking a toll on our well-being. Scientists who study the multitasking brain are finding that doing more than one thing at a time actually makes us feel less like a productivity superstar and more like a failure. The truth is that it's impossible to fully focus on more than one task at a time; our brains just don't work like that. Studies show that dividing our attention can overload the brain and reduce productivity by as much as 40 percent (and when it comes to dialing while driving, the negative potential is much worse).

Mindfulness, defined most simply as "clear awareness" or "genuine presence," is a way off of the multitasking hamster wheel. When you are mindful, you are fully in the here and now, keenly aware of your mind, body, and environment. Mindfulness is a moment-by-moment practice that you can implement any time of the day or night and during any activity (or non-activity). If you're washing the dishes mindfully, you are doing nothing more than washing dishes. You're feeling the warm, soapy water running between your fingers, noticing the weight of the plates and glasses in your hands. You're not daydreaming about what you're going to do this weekend or replaying an argument you had with your spouse. The same formula is applied when playing with a young child, meeting with a colleague at work, or reading this book. When you implement mindfulness you are fully engaged in whatever you are doing—consider it *monotasking*. Cultivating this skill will help to reduce brain overload and will actually help you tackle each task with more efficiency by training your brain to focus on doing one thing really well.

Mindfulness will also be your ally as we move deeper into the era of the selfie and the status update. It is extraordinarily difficult to remain present with what's happening right in front of you when there is intense pressure to remain constantly connected and plugged in. These days we always seem to have one foot outside of our experiences, posting photos of our friends instead of talking to them, taking stylized pictures of our food when we dine out, and fact-checking dinner party observations made by our table mates. Social media is the archenemy of the present moment: Each time you lower your eyes to your device, you essentially leave the room, breaking human connection and adding more tasks to your brain's already overflowing list. Now you also have to come up with 140 witty characters, choose the right filter for that sunset photo, and stalk Snapchat to see what your ex-boyfriend is up to these days. In choosing to be mindful, you create healthy boundaries by committing to doing just one thing at a time and, in doing so, giving yourself the gift of sinking into everything the present moment has to offer.

There's another bonus to this practice. With time, mindfulness helps you begin to develop clearer awareness of your inner experience, in particular the dance of emotions and the swirl of urges that spur unhelpful actions like reaching for a treat, drink, or cigarette when under stress. Awareness, as simple as it seems, is the first step in loosening the grip of those habits. With awareness, you can notice the craving but choose not to act on it; with awareness, you can even notice the thoughts and beliefs surrounding the urge—like that you *need* that cookie or cigarette to calm down. You now have a small space to look at that belief and ask if it's true—rather than let it be a controlling trigger.

HOW TO PRACTICE

Mindfulness is an ongoing practice, a moment-by-moment decision to be exactly where you are right now. You can choose to be mindful at any moment of your day. Why not start now? Feel the weight of this book in your hands (or feel your device if you've chosen to read electronically, but stay with this book—no social media!), notice your butt on the chair, see the words on the page, sense the temperature of the room. Whenever in doubt, simply follow your senses to quickly and easily click into mindfulness: What do you see, feel, taste, hear, smell in this exact moment? Remember to notice the rise and fall of your breath—your pathway into presence. When you're tapped into your senses, you are mindful and present. This is something you can practice anytime, anywhere.

>>

Doing multiple things at once may seem like a normal, even practical approach to managing a busy life, but this relentless juggling of tasks is taking a toll on our well-being.

<<

WHY MEDITATE?

ONCE AN ESOTERIC PRACTICE RESERVED FOR YOGIS AND MONKS, MEDITATION HAS MADE ITS WAY INTO THE MAINSTREAM. MEDITATION APPS ARE A BIG HIT ON SMARTPHONES, BRIGHT AND MODERN MEDITATION STUDIOS ARE AVAILABLE FOR DROP-IN SESSIONS ALL ACROSS THE COUNTRY, AND IT'S NOT UNCOMMON TO SEE SOMEONE

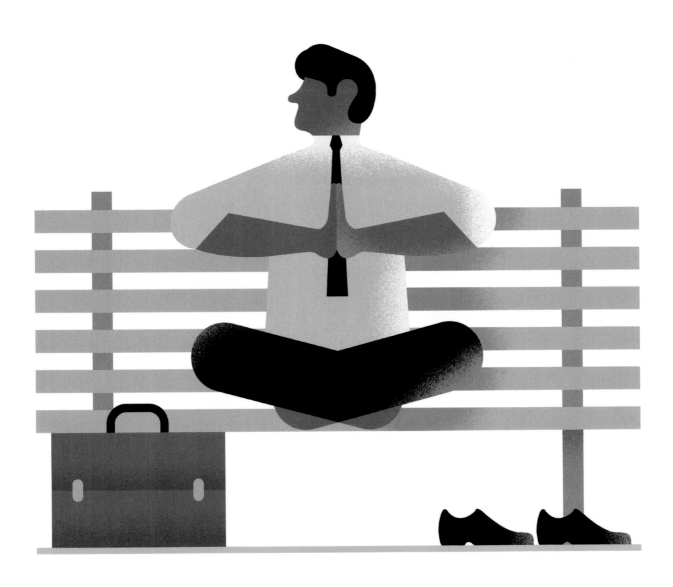

MEDITATING ON THE SUBWAY OR ON A PARK BENCH (no, they're not sleeping).

Like mindfulness, meditation is an essential ally that can help you manage the pressures of contemporary living. Consistent meditators understand that the value of the practice is not so much about reaching some vaulted state of nirvana or enlightenment, but about reaping the benefits that become apparent when they're not meditating. Meditation cultivates adaptability and resilience and reduces reactivity. A steady practice can help you manage strong emotions and ride the choppy waves of life, whether that looks like an angry teenager, a demanding boss, bumper-to-bumper traffic, or anything in between. A regular meditation practice helps create a foundation from which you can never be fully rocked.

There is also a growing field of research on the physiological benefits. The practice has a remarkably positive influence on the brain, helping to improve attention, memory, processing speed, and creativity, and it may even counteract the age-related atrophying that can lead to cognitive conditions like dementia. Meditating is also linked to decreased blood pressure and reduced stress and anxiety, which is why a daily practice "primes the pump" for easier sleep onset at night. Thankfully, you don't need to commit to a month-long silent retreat to reap the enormous benefits of the practice. Regular sitting for as little as ten minutes a day can have positive effects. As for learning how to meditate, there are many options available: apps like Headspace and Calm, books by established teachers, and even YouTube demonstrations, but nothing beats working directly with an instructor. Although books and apps are a good introduction, it's easy to get discouraged and give up if you feel you're not succeeding. Building a relationship with a teacher will help you develop and maintain a lifelong practice.

 HOW TO BE WELL EXPERT I asked **Lodro Rinzler**, a friend and Chief Spiritual Officer of MNDFL Meditation, a meditation studio with three locations in New York City, to answer four common questions about meditation.

1. **THERE SEEM TO BE SO MANY MEDITATION STYLES** out there, from ancient techniques to modern apps. How do I know which one to pick? Do some people "shop around"?

    It's a bit like a musical instrument. I recommend trying a few out, seeing which you really connect to, and then going deep with that. But the "shop around" period is important! The one thing I always recommend is making sure you're studying with trained and certified teachers, who have learned a technique from a teacher who studied with a teacher and on and on back hundreds, if not thousands, of years. Often in the West, when we talk about meditation, we're either talking about time-tested techniques that stem from the Vedas, a five-thousand-year-old oral tradition of mantra-based meditation, or my tradition, Buddhism, which dates back 2,600 years. Perhaps the most well-known practice within Buddhism is mindfulness of the breath, which is a particularly potent technique for anyone looking to be more present with their day-to-day life.

2. **ONCE I'VE PICKED A STYLE TO TRY, HOW DO I BEGIN?** What is the strategy to develop an ongoing practice?

    Once you learn a practice, consistency is probably the most important component to really get going: a consistent type of meditation, consistent amount of time you do it, consistent time of day, consistent environment in your home, and consistent pacing (taking the time to do it every day until it becomes a habit). Taking ten minutes a day to bring your full attention to your breath is a great beginning. We all have to start somewhere!

3. **WHAT ARE REALISTIC EXPECTATIONS TO HAVE ABOUT MEDITATING?** Should I expect to "go deep" and find lasting peace and enlightenment?

    Meditation takes longer than we'd like it to when it comes to seeing the effects. We do become less stressed out, more productive, better sleepers, and

Meditation is an essential ally that can help you manage the pressures of contemporary living.

more, but it takes training and time. In the same way that you wouldn't go to the gym once and expect to lose ten pounds, you can't meditate once and feel forever peaceful. But in both situations, the more you do it, the more you see the results. Along those lines, the biggest misconception about meditation may be that we should be able to sit down and turn the mind off. That would be like asking the heart to stop beating (which would be equally hard to do). We have between sixty thousand to eighty thousand thoughts a day. So it's a good idea to expect that thoughts will come up and to think of meditation as a way to become familiar with your mental landscape. The more we do that, the more we befriend and ultimately learn to love ourselves.

4. WHAT KIND OF SUPPORT IS OUT THERE FOR MODERN-DAY MEDITATORS who really want an ongoing practice, but need a bit of help?

I always recommend working with a teacher, either in a group setting or one on one. Having someone in-person is great, so they get to know you and can help you with your posture, keep track of your journey, and more. Going to a class helps hold us accountable, and nothing beats the energy of sitting shoulder to shoulder with a number of people who are doing the same practice you are. That's a big part of why we founded MNDFL, to make meditation as accessible as possible. For people who don't live near a meditation studio there are Buddhist centers around the world (I recommend Shambhala) and online platforms; you can even take classes with me and other teachers I recommend via MNDFL Video (mndflmeditation. com).I also recommend the pragmatic technique of Vedic meditation, which helps the body release stress and drop into a state of deep restfulness, and is a favorite of the Be Well team. Meet the teachers at vedicmeditation.net.

JUST SAY **NO**

IN OUR OVERCOMMITTED, OVERWORKED, OFTEN OVERWHELMING DAY-TO-DAY EXISTENCE, THERE IS GREAT POWER IN A TINY WORD: NO. THIS ONE SYLLABLE CAN HAVE A BIG IMPACT WHEN—AND IF—IT ACTUALLY ESCAPES FROM YOUR LIPS. SAYING NO IS EASIER SAID THAN DONE AS WE ARE INCESSANTLY ASKED TO SHOW

UP FOR PROFESSIONAL AND FAMILY OBLIGATIONS and always working to be the best employee, parent, spouse, friend, and neighbor (not to mention always being available to others thanks to technology). We tell ourselves that we have to deliver at top level no matter what and too often feel obligated to show up for everyone who reaches out to us. These goals are beyond aspirational—they're simply unreachable—and as you stretch yourself to unimaginable lengths something must get sacrificed. If you put too much on one plate, it's guaranteed to spill over, and usually what gets sacrificed is your own well-being. Things like rest, exercise, personal restoration, and connection, as well as healthy food, get pushed aside as we strive to dig up reserves of the most precious commodity: time.

The pervasive overcommitting that plagues our society is not without consequence. Terms like "burnout" and "chronic exhaustion" are becoming commonplace. Seemingly healthy, vibrant people are hit with stress-induced conditions like shingles and IBS, and some are even hospitalized when they break down mentally and physically from the intense pressure of their lives. The good news is that you are the one who controls how you much you take on. Though at first it can feel challenging,

even scary, to say no, setting limits is a preventative step to protect your well-being and a definitive way to advocate for yourself in a world that will ask you to give until your well has run completely dry.

When you say no, it's like you are drawing a protective force field around yourself and what you have to offer. Knowing when to do this requires paying attention to the red flags your body and mind might be flying in a desperate cry for help. If you are feeling deeply fatigued or depleted, you may have to decline social invitations so you can get to bed early or recharge with a good book or hot bath. You may have to opt out of that extra project at work or that volunteer shift at your child's school that would make you look superhuman. You're not superhuman, you're a regular human like the rest of us and you can do only so much before you short-circuit.

Saying no takes practice. You'll have to accept that you may not always be the most liked or most valued, but in the long run, those who really count will see that it's a strategic part of a self-care regimen and won't take it personally.

The pervasive overcommitting that plagues our society is not without consequence.

ADD REST TO YOUR
WELL-BEING TO-DO LIST

TODAY WE'RE BUSY TO AN ALMOST PATHOLOGICAL DEGREE, FILLING OUR DAYS TO THE BRIM, FILLING OUR MINDS WITH NEWS AND IDEAS, AND FILLING MULTIPLE ROLES AT ONCE, BOTH AT WORK AND AT HOME, IN WAYS OUR PREDECESSORS NEVER DID. THIS NONSTOP STRIVING AND DOING IS REPRESENTATIVE OF OUR

DECIDEDLY *YANG* CULTURE, ONE THAT PRIDES GOING, producing, succeeding, and forcing over softer, slower, more internal *yin* qualities like resting, receiving, and restoring. To live in harmony as a society and in our own bodies, we must strike a balance between the two, just like the yin-yang symbol itself.

In a time when a fundamental biological need like sleep is often pushed to the bottom of our priority list, the idea of blocking out a period of rest during the day can seem downright preposterous. Consciously slowing down to give the body an opportunity to renew and recharge may be unheard of in today's go-go-go society, but intentional rest is the essential counterbalance to all of this action. Most people view rest as a luxury they can't afford or something reserved for the lazy or unambitious. But slowing down, whether through self-care rituals like taking a bath, attending a yoga class, or walking in nature, or by planning regular vacations, is an essential part of a balanced system of health and well-being.

I've found that it helps the buzzing Western mind to frame this downtime as "deliberate rest." You're not doing nothing when you give yourself a restorative break. You're giving your body a chance to rebuild resilience, return to homeostasis, and get back in tune with its natural rhythms. Deliberate rest is not empty, wasted time. On the contrary, these restorative pockets allow you to refuel and prepare for the next burst of productivity and avoid falling into the trap of another of our modern conditions: burnout. If you view your life as a trampoline, periods of conscious rest are like the moment before you're launched back into the air. What goes up must come down.

Rest doesn't look one particular way, and what may feel restorative to one person may feel jarring to another. You may choose to meditate, knit, hike, or spend time with a close friend. The only guidelines to consider when factoring deliberate rest into your life are to stick to your commitment to give yourself this downtime, as it can be all too easy to push it aside for other obligations, and to make an effort to truly give your mind and body a break. For many this will mean dropping all devices—real downtime won't come from cruising Tumblr or binging on Netflix shows.

>> **When you are subjected to ongoing mental and physical demands but deprived of rest and recovery, your whole nervous system takes a toll.** <<

>>

You're not doing nothing when you give yourself a restorative break. You're giving your body a chance to rebuild resilience, return to homeostasis, and get back in tune with its natural rhythms.

<<

HOW TO REST

It may seem strange, but many of us need to learn, or relearn, how to rest. The first step is factoring rest into your day. Like most things that you want to accomplish, you'll have to plan your period of rest. As you review your day in the morning, see where you can add in at least ten minutes of deliberate rest. This can be a short walk outside, a brief meditation, or a breathing exercise (page 184). Consider the four types of active rest (as opposed to sleep, which is passive rest) as defined by Matthew Edlund, MD, in his book *The Power of Rest:*

PHYSICAL REST: breathing techniques, restorative yoga, taking a hot bath

MENTAL REST: meditation, visualizations, mindful walking in nature, listening to music

SOCIAL REST: spending time with people who make you feel good

SPIRITUAL REST: prayer, spending time in nature, connecting with things greater than yourself

Take a moment to see which category you do the least, and think about how and where you could drop a few minutes of this into your day, today, and every day this week.

GIVE YOURSELF A MASSAGE

SELF-MASSAGE IS A SIMPLE AND IMPACTFUL ACT OF SELF-CARE THAT IS AFFORDABLE, DOABLE, AND DEEPLY RESTORATIVE. I'M PARTIAL TO ABHYANGA, WHICH IS AN AYURVEDIC OIL MASSAGE. THIS ANCIENT STRESS-RELIEVING TREATMENT DOUBLES AS AN EASY ACT OF MINDFULNESS: YOU CAN PRACTICE BECOMING DEEPLY

PRESENT WITH THE SENSORY EXPERIENCE OF TOUCH on your body.

Abhyanga also brings mental, emotional, and physical balance. Regular practice can improve muscle tone, increase circulation, calm the nervous system, and assist the lymph in detoxification—it's considered a purifying treatment in India. It uses long, fluid strokes that are said to activate and clear the energy meridians of the body, and the abundance of warm oils has a grounding and lubricating effect (similar to eating healthy fats and oils), which is why it also feels so good.

You can use warm sesame, almond, or coconut oil (pick the best quality you can, as, in a sense, your skin "eats" the oils). In summer, coconut has a cooling effect; in fall and winter, sesame has a warming effect. A practice of Abhyanga can help connect you to the seasons (page 242). In particular, it can balance out the raw, edgy sensations you can feel at the onset of cold, windy weather, helping you feel more nurtured and grounded. Learning your dominant "dosha," or energy type, can help you pick the oil that suits you best for the most effective soothing; dosha quizzes are easy to find online. The key, according to Ayurvedic teaching, is to leave the oil on for at least seven and a half minutes so it can saturate the skin.

>>

Meditation, mindfulness, breath work, and soothing touch are not luxurious extras, they are daily essentials for managing imbalance and maintaining the body's healing power.

HERE'S HOW TO GIVE YOURSELF AN ABHYANGA MASSAGE:

STEP 1 Warm the oil by running hot water over the bottle (if plastic) or setting it in a pan of hot water (if glass). Test the temperature on your inner wrist; it should be pleasingly warm, not hot.

STEP 2 Pour a quarter-sized amount of oil into your palm and apply it to the crown of your head. Using circular strokes, massage your entire scalp. Then, using a circular motion, massage your face, using an upward motion across your forehead, temples, cheeks, jaws, ears, and earlobes.

STEP 3 Move to your arms and legs, adding more oil as needed, and using long upward strokes, always in the direction of your heart. Use a circular motion on your elbows and knees.

STEP 4 Move to your belly. Massage along the path of your large intestine, moving in circular strokes up the right side of your abdomen, across it, and down the left side, then focusing your touch on the circle immediately around the navel (where tension is often stored). You can use both hands to stroke your sides and lower back, too. Then massage your chest in large circular strokes.

STEP 5 Finally, massage each foot for a few dedicated minutes, getting into the soles and each of the toes.

STEP 6 Leave the oil on your body for up to fifteen minutes so it can sink in. Use this time to meditate or deeply relax. Then take a warm bath or shower without scrubbing and soaping, or over-shampooing your hair. Afterward, towel-dry gently.

Note: If you don't have time to give yourself the full-body treatment, focus on your scalp, ears, navel, palms, and the soles of your feet.

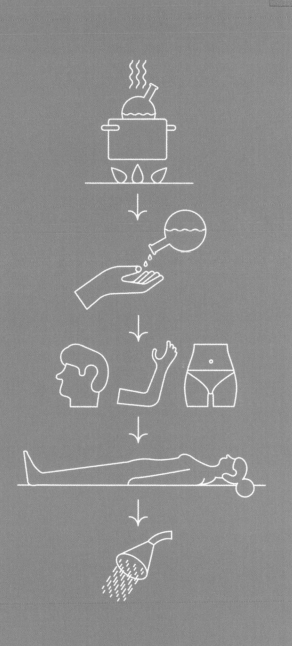

GET HANDY

WHEN WAS THE LAST TIME YOU MADE SOMETHING WITH YOUR HANDS? WE ARE SENSORY BEINGS, NATURALLY DESIGNED TO USE OUR EYES AND OUR HANDS TO CREATE, BUT AS WE AGE WE GET FURTHER AWAY FROM THE FREE-FORM FINGER PAINTING AND CRAYON DRAWINGS OF OUR YOUTH AND DEEPER INTO OUR OWN HEADS.

MOST ADULTS LIVE ENTIRELY IN THE WORLD OF THE mind, forgetting how good it feels to get messy and creative by drawing, sculpting, or sewing. Getting crafty isn't only fun and satisfying—it feels great to make something out of nothing—it has health benefits as well. Studies are finding a direct link between artistic activities and reduced levels of cortisol (the stress hormone). Some crafting activities can be calming, meditative even, and may even launch you into an entirely different mental space, where creativity flows and perfection takes a backseat.

Doing something with your hands can also free up your mind to focus. Many people knit while listening to lectures or watching informative videos. Creative pursuits can also have a community aspect: Knitting and sewing circles abound as activities that were once reserved for your grandma are experiencing a renaissance as younger generations tap into the pleasure of DIY endeavors. This is seen in the explosion of Etsy's handcrafted online shops and the ever-expanding Maker movement, where it is extremely cool to fabricate your own robots, machines, and board games. There are even places like DIY Bar in Portland, Oregon, where you can sip craft beers and meet new people while tackling leatherworking and jewelry-making projects.

You don't have to have prior experience or genuine artistic talent to tap into the benefits of artistic expression, and there are many different avenues to pursue. The next time you feel the need to decompress and long to create something that's entirely yours, check out these easy crafting ideas. (You can find instructions online; YouTube is particularly helpful.)

1. MAKE HOMEMADE PLAY DOUGH

2. KNIT A SCARF OR A HAT

3. CREATE A SIMPLE QUILT

4. DIG INTO ADULT COLORING BOOKS (there are incredibly detailed and dynamic options available today)

5. GET MESSY WITH A FINGER PAINTING SESSION

6. PRACTICE ORIGAMI (YouTube is a wonderful resource for the beginning paper sculptor)

7. TURN ON YOUR INNER ARCHITECT with an ice pop stick house

8. DESIGN A CUSTOMIZED MOBILE using sticks, twine, rocks, feathers, leaves, or anything else that strikes your fancy

9. USE PINTEREST TO IGNITE SOME PAPER CHAIN INSPIRATION—they can be more sophisticated than you think

10. COLLECT SAND AT YOUR NEXT BEACH VISIT, tint it with vibrant colors, and layer it in glass bottles for beautiful sand art

Once a habit is developed, it works effortlessly for you, partly because the brain loves habits. When lifestyle choices become habitual, they are automatic.

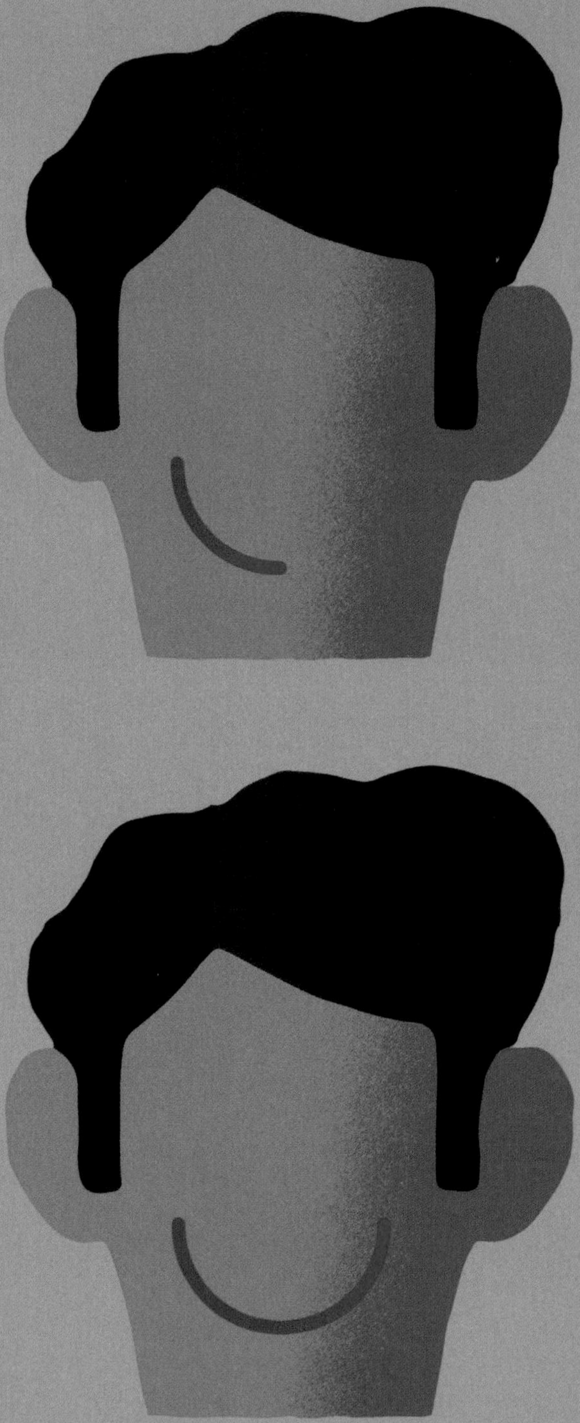

SMILE. **LAUGH.** REPEAT.

YOU MAKE AN EFFORT TO INCLUDE EXERCISE AND vegetables into your daily life, but do you make sure to include laughter, too? Regular chuckles really are great medicine, helping to lower blood pressure and cortisol levels, decrease pain, and even stabilize blood sugar. Researchers have also found that laughter stimulates chemical changes in the brain that help protect us against the harmful effects of chronic stress.

When you laugh you're stimulating the release of endorphins, the happy brain chemicals that are released after a good workout. Giggles also help reduce inflammation; release tension in the muscles of the face, neck, shoulders, and abdomen; and fight viruses and tumors by giving the immune system a welcome boost. You'll even rev your metabolism with a few minutes of joyful guffaws. It's like taking your medicine, only funnier.

You can factor laughter into your day by listening to stand-up comedy or a funny podcast in your kitchen as you prep food and then clean all the dishes, or on your commute. Invite a friend or loved one to share a half-hour of a laugh-inducing show (comedic news shows fronted by hosts like John Oliver, Stephen Colbert, Trevor Noah, and Samantha Bee have a knack for finding the funny in increasingly disheartening times). Even just a skit or two from *Saturday Night Live* or Funny or Die can punctuate your day with a humorous exclamation point. Just resist the temptation to watch this stuff in the wee hours—catch up on what you missed the next day so you don't disrupt your sleep!

WHEN IT COMES TO GETTING A DAILY DOSE of laughter, podcasts give you an array and diversity of talent that exceeds anything network and cable networks can offer, especially given that you can get your laughs from around the globe. Find a few voices you click with and subscribe to their podcasts, and they will keep you regularly updated with new episodes. From the cult-favorite TV recap show *Bitch Sesh* or unconventional chat shows *With Special Guest Lauren Lapkus*, *WTF with Marc Maron*, *Anna Faris Is Unqualified*, and *2 Dope Queens*, to the freeform-style *improv4humans* and comedian meet-up *Don't Get Me Started*—and many, many more, once you start looking—you can curate a humor fix that fits your personal funny bone.

Laughter stimulates chemical changes in the brain that help protect us against the harmful effects of stress.

◀◀

OPEN THE GATES TO TRANQUILITY: 3 YOGA POSES TO CALM AND RESTORE

YOGA CAN STRENGTHEN AND ENERGIZE. IT CAN ALSO BE AN EFFECTIVE ROUTE TO A QUIETER MIND AND A CALMER NERVOUS SYSTEM. YOU DON'T HAVE TO BE AN EXPERIENCED YOGI OR IN TOP PHYSICAL FORM TO

TAP INTO THE BENEFITS OF YOGA'S GENTLER SIDE. Yin yoga or restorative yoga can be utilized by those at all fitness levels to reset and recalibrate the body, mind, and spirit.

This is not the fast-paced yoga that you see in typical hatha or vinyasa classes, where you bop between poses with a mere breath between each. Restorative poses are designed to be held for longer periods of time to allow your muscles to soften and your busy mind to become still. Simple props like bolsters, blankets, blocks, or a chair support you while you let go of tension held deep within the musculoskeletal system—they mold you into shapes that open up space within your body. Lying over a bolster, for instance, benefits the lungs and heart. In addition, props help you remain in a pose long enough for the benefits to take effect and your mind to begin to slow and quiet.

This slower-paced yoga triggers the parasympathetic nervous system, causing your flight-or-fight stress response (the same reaction you'd have to seeing a bear in the woods) to fall away. In this tension-free place, you'll experience an expansiveness that will allow you to let go: Your muscles soften, your breathing slows, and your bones release at the joints. When you transition (slowly! deliberately!) out of each posture and into the next, you'll have a newfound sense of how your body moves.

3 SIMPLE RESTORATIVE YOGA POSES

Setting up each restorative pose is a key part of this practice. The idea is to design the ultimate support system for full release.

CHAIR CROSS-LEGGED FORWARD BEND

BENEFITS: This modified forward bend allows you to reap the benefits of the pose without overextending your hamstrings or lower back. It releases tension in the shoulders and neck while calming the nerves and reducing stress.

Sit cross-legged on a bolster or two folded blankets with a chair in front of you. Place a folded blanket on the chair seat. Extend forward and rest your forehead on the chair. Fold your arms and place them on the chair seat above your head. Hold the pose for five to ten minutes, reversing the cross of your legs halfway through.

RECLINING CROSS-LEGGED POSE

BENEFITS: This pose gives a gentle stretch to the inner thighs, groin, and knees; stimulates the heart and improves circulation; and helps reduce stress, mild depression, and the uncomfortable symptoms of menstruation and menopause.

Sit cross-legged and place a bolster or three firmly folded blankets vertically behind you, a few inches away from your sacrum. (If you are using a yoga mat, this support will run vertically up the center.) Lie back onto it and place a large blanket folded in thirds under your head to support it; your head should be higher than your heart and tilted so that your chin is lower than your forehead. The body is in a gentle sloping position in this pose, with the head above the heart and the heart above the pelvis. If your hips are tight, place folded blankets under each thigh so you can fully sink into the pose, with no pulling on your inner thighs. Let your arms fall outward at the sides of your body, with the backs of your hands resting lightly on the floor. When you have found the right combination of support, you will be able to easily relax your face and throat and feel as if you are safely held. Notice your breath as it moves in and out of your lungs. Remain in the pose for ten minutes, changing the cross of the legs halfway through.

INVERSION: LEGS UP THE WALL

BENEFITS: This pose is especially wonderful if you've been on your feet for hours. It helps relieve swollen ankles and varicose veins, reduces mild back pain, zaps anxiety, and even helps alleviate mild depression and insomnia. Turning upside down is a wonderful way to reboot and recharge.

Place the short side of a yoga mat against a wall, then put a bolster or three firmly folded blankets on the mat a few inches from the wall. Kneel to the side of the mat, facing away from the wall. Lean sideways over the bolster, pivot your hips, and swing your legs up the wall. Rest your pelvis on the bolster and your sit bones and heels against the wall. The back of your head and the tops of your shoulders should be sinking into the mat while you hold up your legs vertically. Your arms should be turned out at the sockets, resting comfortably at your sides with your hands and wrists relaxed. Feel your lumbar spine releasing and spreading from the center to the sides. Soften the sockets of your eyes, feeling the body release tension from the skull down to the heart. Remain in the pose for five to fifteen minutes.

When you are ready to come out of the pose, bend your legs and push your feet against the wall to slide off the bolster. Then bend your knees to your chest and roll over onto your right side before slowly pushing yourself up, rolling your head up last.

Restorative poses are designed to be held for longer periods of time to allow your muscles to soften and your busy mind to become still.

LET GO AND FORGIVE

THOUGH HOLDING GRUDGES IS RARELY INCLUDED IN A LIST OF POSSIBLE FACTORS CONTRIBUTING TO COMPROMISED HEALTH, I BELIEVE THAT STOCKPILING EMOTIONAL PAIN CAN HAVE A SERIOUS IMPACT ON OUR WELL-BEING, AND I'M NOT ALONE. DOCTORS AT THE MOOD DISORDERS ADULT CONSULTATION CLINIC AT

THE JOHNS HOPKINS HOSPITAL HAVE FOUND THAT there is a direct correlation between the hurt and disappointment we carry and our state of wellness. Emotions like anger and resentment trigger our fight-or-flight response, activating changes in our heart rate, blood pressure, and immune response. Forgiveness, on the other hand, reduces stress and anxiety and calms the nervous system, which can help us remain healthy.

For me, the essential role that forgiveness plays in our human experience rose to the surface after I had the great honor of meeting Archbishop Desmond Tutu. I believe he is the human representation of forgiveness, and our conversations have remained with me to this day. He explained that forgiveness is not about disregarding the offense you experienced at the hand of another, but about liberating yourself from the steely grip of anger. The archbishop reminded me that when you forgive, you are liberating yourself from the rage or resentment churning within you. In forgiving, you release yourself.

Forgiving is a process that won't happen overnight. The journey begins by first allowing yourself to fully feel your pain. Reaching out to a friend or therapist can help give your hurt space to move through you. Then, when you feel ready, you can start to flip your perspective by imagining what it would feel like to be the person who hurt you: How had his or her life unfolded up to the point of the pain? In doing this you are not exonerating their actions, you're simply trying to connect to their experience as another human being. This may lead you to compassion and then to forgiveness.

Forgiving yourself is also essential. We all make mistakes, even big ones. In fact, mistakes are the primary way we learn, so consider your errors part of your education in becoming a better human being. And take special note of what some Buddhists call "the second arrow," that extra poke we give ourselves after messing up. The mistake was enough. Don't add to your pain by also pointing a second arrow at your heart.

A NEW APPROACH TO LETTING GO

The practice of Radical Honesty is a communication technique designed to promote authenticity, intimacy, and personal growth, and that can help you move beyond past hurts and create a healthier way through conflict. It sees honesty as key to both intimacy and forgiveness because real connection is based on honestly sharing what is true for you. Honesty Lab, a new facilitator of this well-known practice, offers in-person workshops around the country as well as online courses and remote coaching. Says founder John Rosania, "There is a difference between full-bodied forgiveness and mental forgiveness. The first is an experience of actual change and release in the body that brings about a wave of actual forgiveness and appreciation. Sensations in the body change, and when they do, thoughts change. The second is what most people mean by forgiveness, which is a willed mental act: 'You should forgive your parents so you can move on.' The first is very powerful and rooted in honesty, the second is play acting." Discover more about them at honesty-lab.com.

PLAY FOOTSIE
WITH A TENNIS BALL

IF YOU HAVE ACCESS TO A TENNIS BALL, YOU HAVE ACCESS TO ONE OF THE EASIEST METHODS OF TENSION-
RELEASE AVAILABLE. OUR FEET HAVE A BIG JOB TO DO, CARRYING US WHERE WE NEED TO GO, OFTEN IN
SHOES THAT ARE NOT THE BEST FIT FOR THE TASK. GIVING THEM A BIT OF FOCUSED ATTENTION FOR FIVE TO

TEN MINUTES A DAY CAN HAVE EFFECTS THAT RIPPLE out to the rest of the body, and you can do it anywhere, like under your desk at work or while standing at the kitchen counter prepping dinner.

Rolling a tennis ball under each foot is a direct route to a targeted fascia release (page 137). It's a simple acupressure technique that releases tight muscles and fascia in the feet, which reduces strain and pressure on the toes and toe joints, which in turn improves balance and stimulates stress relief and well-being throughout the entire body. Notice how just three to five minutes of rolling allows your heart rate to slow, your breath to open, and a satisfying stillness to take over.

HERE'S HOW TO DO IT:

STEP 1 Stand on a surface with a bit of friction, like a carpeted floor or a yoga mat. Place a tennis ball under the arch of one foot and ease the weight of your body onto the ball.

STEP 2 Alternate slowly flexing your toes over the ball and then clenching them like a fist. Repeat five times, then move the ball to a different part of your foot.

STEP 3 When you find a tender spot on your foot, apply as much pressure as you can handle and hold for a few seconds. Then find the next area of tenderness and hold. Continue until you have visited every area of your foot.

STEP 4 After you finish the first foot, stand with both feet on the floor and note the difference between them—it should be notable. Switch to the other foot and repeat.

Note: This process will be painful in spots. This is normal, but if you feel pain that is particularly sharp, move to another area.

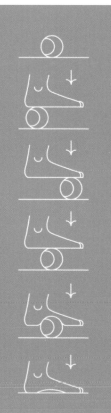

SEXUAL HEALING

SEX IS ONE OF THE MOST EFFECTIVE—AND FREE—WELLNESS TECHNIQUES AVAILABLE TO HUMANKIND. OFTEN OVERLOOKED OR FORGOTTEN, ESPECIALLY AS WE GET OLDER, THE SIMPLE ACT OF PLEASURE HAS AN EVER-GROWING LINEUP OF HEALTH BENEFITS THAT'S DIFFICULT TO IGNORE. YET PUSHING SEX TO THE TOP OF YOUR

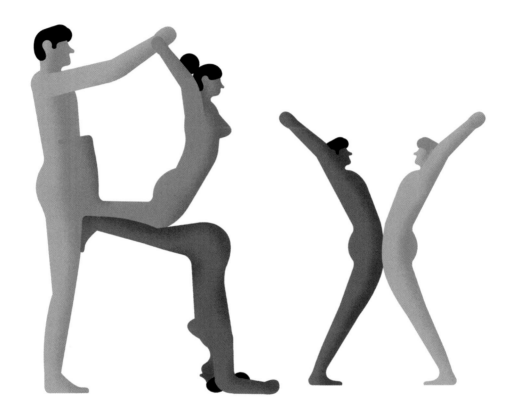

PRIORITY LIST CAN FEEL CHALLENGING. IF YOU, LIKE many modern humans, feel like your sex drive has slumped, the first thing to look at is sleep deprivation. Lack of sleep is the biggest passion killer out there because, from your body's point of view, when you're deprived of the energy necessary for survival tasks, nonessential extras like pleasurable sex get the back, back seat. (Conversely, when you're deeply rested, your desire and orgasmic potential typically surge.)

The second area to look at is movement: Find a movement practice that moves you (page 119), and notice how it wakes up a new sensitivity to your body and its healthful urges. The third area is your own tendency to prioritize productivity over intimacy and sensuality. Only you can reevaluate that, but I encourage you to push past the intoxicating pull of to-dos and make time for sex, whether the kind with a partner or solo self-enjoyment. Do it regularly, and you'll find that your relationship or sense of self-love becomes stronger, your skin brighter, and your disposition sunnier. You'll be healthier *and* happier.

SEX IS:

STRESS REDUCING. Angry, anxious, worried, or overwhelmed? Channel that restless mental energy into something more positive: boudoir play. Chances are high you'll feel better on the other side.

IMMUNE ENHANCING. Nookie on the regular helps keep your immune system in tip-top shape. Notice that those who get some often are rarely sniffling and sneezing.

ENERGY BURNING. An average romp is comparable to a modest workout on a treadmill—and it's a lot more fun.

SLEEP SUPPORTING. A good session will trigger sleep-inducing endorphins that will carry you off to dreamland.

INCONTINENCE BUSTING. Sex tones the pelvic muscles that support your uterus, bladder, and bowels, leading to better urinary control.

AGE DEFYING. Trade the Botox for some booty. An active sex life promotes the release of hormones like testosterone and estrogen, which slows the aging process and keeps the body looking young and vital. Regular sex also gives your skin a healthy glow that will last way beyond the post-coital cuddle by increasing blood circulation, which pumps more oxygen to the skin, resulting in a brighter appearance. Sex also boosts our natural collagen production, which helps to prevent age spots and sagging.

PAIN RELIEVING. You might change "Not tonight, honey, I have a headache" to "Yes tonight, honey, I have a headache." The hormone oxytocin is secreted in your body through sexual arousal and orgasm, which in turn causes the release of endorphins that act as a powerful analgesic.

CONFIDENCE BOOSTING. When you show up in the bedroom, it's easier to show up for the rest of your life. Pleasing your partner while also having your own desires fulfilled is a surefire method of increasing your self-esteem. You can then bring that mojo to client meetings, creative undertakings, and interactions with family and friends.

ADVICE ON MAKING SEX A BETTER experience is in no shortage if you subscribe to glossy magazines, but there are other ways to get information. One of these is OMGYes.com, a refreshingly frank and informative website devoted to the "science of pleasure." It empowers women—and their partners—with pragmatic knowledge about achieving and enhancing orgasm.

HAPPY MAKING. Sex makes you happier than having money. According to a recent study by the National Bureau of Economic Research, a marriage that included regular humping was figured to bring the same levels of happiness as earning an extra $100,000 annually.

If you feel like your sex drive has slumped, the first thing to look at is sleep deprivation.

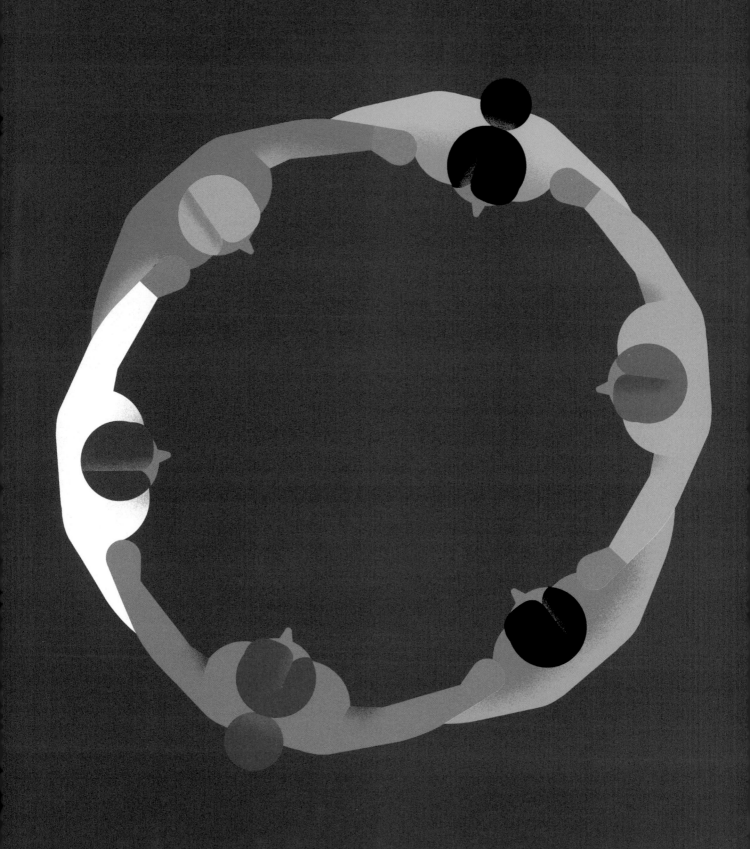

CONNECT

FOR EONS, HUMANS LIVED IN A WEB OF CONNEC-
tivity. We were connected to nature for the resources
of food and shelter; to the seasons and weather, which
dictated daily activities; and most of all to each other as
we lived in interdependent groups in which every member played an important role. Though existence was far
from easy—often it was brutal and harsh—our physiology
evolved in response to cues from nature, and our perspective was shaped by knowing our place in the world.

Today, the pendulum has swung to the other extreme.
We live with fierce independence, cut off from extended
family, insulated from wilderness, and short of leisure
time for friends. Sprawling towns can make community
harder to find, and despite the noise of constant communication, intimacy in a time of fractured attention spans
can be fleeting. It used to be the elderly who were at
risk of loneliness and decline, but now age is no barrier.
You can be young and lonely, or in midlife and struggling
to find meaning. And while Western medicine tends to
brush off these considerations as minor, I see them as
crucial to good health. Invisible things like bonded relationships, a sense of purpose, and a feeling of belonging
are as influential as anything you can measure or test in a
lab. They instill security, confidence, and a healthy sense
of self—qualities that are cornerstones of resilient well-
being and give greater immunity to disease and the many
expressions of stress.

There are three ropes of connection that help to anchor
you in a meaningful life: relationship to the natural world
(the macrocosm that contains you); relationships with a
few people who know you well and see you for who you
are; and the relationship with your own emotional terrain
and all its ebbs and flows. Use the actions in this ring
to enliven these three ropes. Then they will be there for
you, holding you securely, in moments of challenge and
of ease alike.

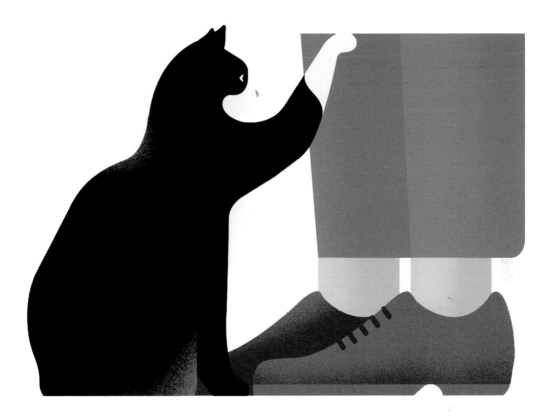

LOVE A PET

WOOF! **OR, IF YOU PREFER,** *MIAOW!* **HAVING AN ANIMAL FRIEND MAY DO MORE FOR YOU THAN ANY SUPER-** FOOD EVER COULD. IN STUDY AFTER STUDY, PET OWNERS ARE HEALTHIER AND HAPPIER THAN NON-PET OWNERS.

CARING FOR A PET DELIVERS MULTIDIMENSIONAL health-boosting effects: lowering stress and boosting cardiovascular health while ensuring you get out for exercise rain or shine (less so for a cat, obviously). Most important, tending to the needs of an animal pays back with an experience of secure attachment to another—it is a relationship of interdependence and unconditional love that nurtures your sense of belonging and feeds your sense of purpose, day in and day out.

Getting a pet is nothing to take lightly—they require your commitment, devotion, playtime, and, for the canine kind, several walks on a daily basis, not to mention food and vet visits. But when it comes to the health of your body, heart, and spirit, what you get in return is priceless. If you can't own a pet, to get a dose of four-footed love in your life, consider volunteering at shelters, fostering for short amounts of time, or offering to walk or care for friends' pets.

Pair up with an animal in need through adoptapet.com, adopt-a-dog.org, or petfinder.com.

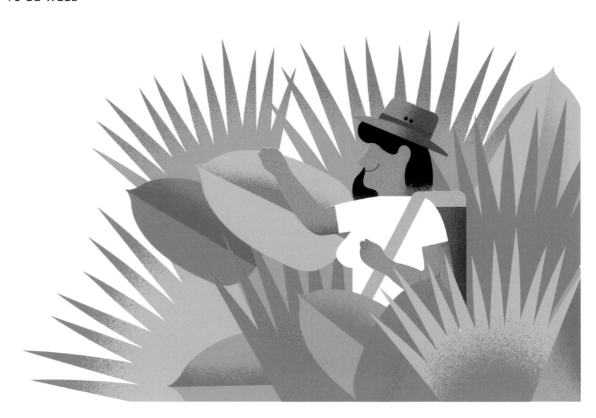

GO WILD
(OR AT LEAST GET OUTSIDE!)

WHEN WE RECOGNIZE THE VIRTUES, THE TALENT, THE BEAUTY OF MOTHER EARTH, SOMETHING IS BORN IN US, SOME KIND OF CONNECTION, LOVE IS BORN. —THICH NHAT HANH

CONSIDER THIS YOUR PRESCRIPTION FOR PARKS. OR trailheads, lakes, or meadows. Spending intentional time in verdant surroundings restores something of your original human condition: a calm body with an optimized immune system, and a brain in a state of restful awareness, alert to surroundings but unencumbered by constant thought. Nature helps you find this state by waking up the five senses—it gently feeds your eyes and ears with stimulation that invites your touch and arouses the olfactory system (so much so that one leading researcher in the field of nature therapy believes that the aromatic chem-

icals released by pine trees are responsible for turning on the powerfully anticancer "killer cells" of your immune system). Allowing yourself moments in nature when you fully absorb its atmosphere, sense by sense, has the tremendous effect of rejuvenating the parts of yourself that get dulled and squelched by everyday demands—it brings you back to yourself. The Harvard T.H. Chan School of Public Health found that adults spend an average of only 5 percent of their day outside; getting into green space, daily if possible and definitely every week, is as vitally important as eating your greens.

In Japan and South Korea, formalized wellness practices exist around these principles. For example, the Japanese practice of *shinrin-yoku* translates as "forest bathing" and involves quietly immersing oneself in the sensory atmosphere of trees to restore well-being and soothe a harried mind. Part physical activity, part natural therapy, it's a powerful and low-cost intervention (and no, you don't have to be naked for this kind of bathing!). Doing nothing in nature but being present to the experience initiates a cascade of beneficial effects: The parasympathetic nervous system switches on, cortisol drops, and the brain's prefrontal cortex—your hard-driving command center—takes a break as you drift into a soft-focus state of awareness. This allows you to shift from information overload to a state of pleasure, let go of negative thought cycles, rejuvenate your mental energy, and even access a wellspring of creativity and concentration.

It's been observed that empathy and altruism also increase after gazing at natural sights; this boost might get even better if you get dirt between your toes. A recent study showed how a strain of soil bacteria increased serotonin—a powerful mood-boosting chemical—in mice, suggesting that touching soil itself might be a factor in elevating mood. Today, "ecotherapy" practitioners in the U.S. are harnessing this potential and using exposure to nature as an alternative therapy for physical and mental suffering, one that is low cost, has no side effects, and often leads to greater social connectivity as kindred spirits literally cross paths in a park or on a trail.

Of course, if your personal predisposition is to get after it in the great outdoors by hiking, biking, or skiing through the elements rather than contemplating them, the benefits are still yours to grab. Exercising in green and wild spaces is shown to trump indoor workouts in terms of lower perceived effort, greater motivation, and higher pleasure levels. (Common sense would tell you this, but now researchers are validating it, too.) Just remember to be present in the environment as you move, keeping distractions to a minimum and letting your senses appreciate every sight, sound, and smell; taking children on these expeditions will ensure you stay present to the details.

As for how much nature is necessary to reap the most benefits, Finnish researchers developing antidotes to depression prescribe several short immersions per week, with a forty-minute walk showing significant benefits to state of mind. Meanwhile, trained forest therapy guides in the U.S. recommend seven contemplative walks in seven weeks to begin your own nature therapy practice. But rejuvenation can also be as simple as a lunch break on a bench in a botanical garden or lounging in a park looking at puffy clouds—two options for time-pressed urbanites.

For the fullest benefits, let iconic nature writer Edward Abbey be your inspiration. He said, "Wilderness is not a luxury but a necessity of the human spirit." Venturing beyond everyday boundaries and entering unexplored wilderness is the deepest form of nature refreshment—one study showed a 50 percent increase in mental performance after three days of backpacking—and it also seems to deliver the most transcendent effect. Wilderness enlivens your very essence when you feel dulled or disenchanted, and reminds you that you are as much a part of the cosmos as the sun, moon, and stars.

HOW TO GET YOUR GREEN ON

- GET ON TRAILS with community groups like Hike it Baby (which organizes free group hikes for parents and caregivers with children), Sierra Club, Outdoor Afro, Latino Outdoors, and the Natural Leaders Network.

- PARTICIPATE IN SHINRIN-YOKU SESSIONS in the U.S. with guides listed at natureandforesttherapy.org.

- VOLUNTEER IN AN URBAN FOOD GARDEN, join a bird-watching club, get involved with an environmental activism and cleanup group, or join a naturalist-led hike or herb walk in your area.

- GO CAMPING in beautiful and unique locations using hipcamp.com, or camp in comfort with tentrr.com, which offers canvas tents on platforms.

COMMIT DAILY
RANDOM ACTS OF KINDNESS

SAY A MEANINGFUL "THANK YOU" TO THE CONDUCTOR ON THE TRAIN. LET THAT OTHER DRIVER CUT IN FRONT OF YOU WITH A CHEERY WAVE. CHECK IN ON YOUR ELDERLY NEIGHBOR AND SHARE A COFFEE AND A LAUGH. SMALL ACTS OF KINDNESS ARE MORE THAN JUST A BOON TO THE RECIPIENT—THEY CREATE A MOMENTARY

CONNECTION BETWEEN YOU AND THE WORLD AT large, an instant of intimacy that supports *you* while bestowing compassion on another.

When you are kind to another person with no expectation of anything in return, you experience the "helper's high"—the pleasure and reward centers of *your* brain light up, as if you received the good deed. Your levels of serotonin rise and cortisol goes down, as does your blood pressure—thanks to the secretion of oxytocin, the love and bonding chemical, which also protects your heart by supporting your cardiovascular system—and your body makes endorphins, the natural painkiller. If you tend toward anxiety, choosing to do a kind act every day has been shown to help: Your mood becomes more positive, your confidence increases, and you feel more satisfied in life. You might get an energy boost, too, a newfound sense of strength and empowerment.

Perhaps the biggest benefit of kindness is that it can shift you out of a single-point perspective, in which it's easy to be consumed by personal problems and obstacles, into a shared experience of life. For that moment or few minutes, you remember that we're all in it together. Kindness is a universal language that crosses perceived boundaries and divides, and it's one of the easiest things to exchange—no backstory, explanation, or complex social

dance required. It also becomes your teacher. When you commit an act of kindness, you are not thinking about the past or worrying about the future; "right now" fills your awareness and anchors you to the present. Furthermore, with your kindness you show another person that they've been *seen*—you affirm they belong here—which, even if your intention was just to make a cup of tea, is a powerful gesture in a time when loneliness is rampant. Compassion and mindfulness go hand in hand.

Make a daily act of unsolicited kindness a health habit. The scale of the act doesn't matter. Surprise someone with an authentic compliment about how they handled something, listen closely to an acquaintance who's in need of being heard, lend a hand to someone you don't normally spend time with, or simply smile and make eye contact, even if you don't feel like it. Do something anonymous and unexpected, like paying the toll of the person behind you, or pick up trash when you see it (an act of kindness to your community and the environment). Kindness is a muscle you can start to flex and that grows the more you use it; it's also contagious, as witnessing acts of kindness stimulates feel-good chemistry in others and inspires similar acts. One random act of kindness at a time, we help each other become more present and connected to each other—and healthier, too.

>> **Make a daily act of unsolicited kindness a health habit.** <<

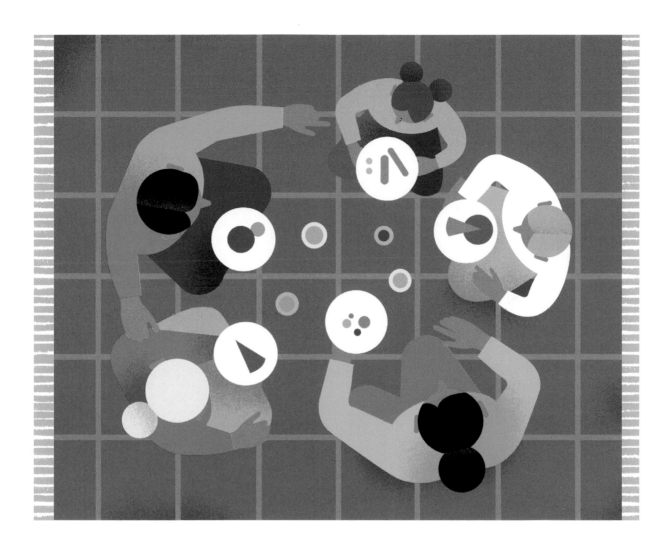

GATHER. EAT. COMMUNE.

GATHERING AROUND A TABLE TO SHARE FOOD WITH OTHERS IS A SIMPLE BUT PROFOUND ACT. YOU MAY ALREADY DO IT, UNCONSCIOUSLY EATING YOUR MEALS WITH FAMILY MEMBERS OR COLLEAGUES AT WORK, OR YOU MAY CONSUME MOST OF YOUR DAILY SUSTENANCE ALONE, QUICKLY, WHILE STANDING AT THE COUNTER

OR WORKING AT YOUR DESK. EITHER WAY, STARTING to bring awareness not only to what you eat, but how (and with whom) you eat is an essential aspect of a well-rounded and happy life.

Since the beginning of time, cooking and eating food with others was an established part of everyday living. Whether it was hunting that evening's meal, preparing and placing it on the fire, and then consuming it as a tribe, or chopping vegetables and meat in the kitchen with siblings, parents, and grandparents and then sharing the soup, sauce, or stew as a family, we are designed to break bread together. Yet, sadly, in this era of constant overworking and hyperconnectivity, meals have been pushed to the sidelines, replaced instead by survivalist eating: sandwiches scarfed in the car, smoothies slurped while racing down the sidewalk, lunches and dinners consumed in front of the computer, TV, or phone. As the family meal fades away, gone with it is the human warmth, joy, and connection that comes from cooking together and sharing food, as well as a balanced and healthy relationship to eating—it's easy to care less about what you're putting into your body when nobody else is watching.

Whether you're the head of a bustling household or you live alone, making time to sit down (the *sitting down* part is key) and share a meal with others on a regular basis will inevitably lead to more peace, stability—and smiles! Human beings are the only animals that ritualize eating and consider the hunger of those who are not family members, and the table is our canvas for this species-specific adaptation. The mealtime table was once the heart of the household, where relatives young and old gathered to connect over the most primal of human needs: feeding ourselves.

The table still plays an essential role, if we choose to use it. The simple flat surface not only holds the food that keeps us fed and nourished (and pleasured when it's delicious), but it also serves as an anchor for our experience as a collective and as individuals. Eating together around the table gives us a set period to check in with each other, serving as a reliable touchstone that adds shape and boundaries to our day and providing space for us to do some necessary downloading. The simple question "How was your day?" invites inquiry and fosters conversation and allows us to release some of what we've experienced. Regular, shared meal times are beneficial for everyone, but kids particularly benefit from a set family dinner. The consistency and connection helps younger kids feel safe and seen and supports older kids in meeting obligations (dinner is at 6:00 each night—don't be late!). Maintaining

a consistent family dinner takes effort, though, so try to sit down together at least three nights a week. The meal itself doesn't have to be restaurant quality; sometimes simply gathering around the table is enough. Give yourself permission to order takeout (ideally, the healthiest you can find!) on particularly busy or long days.

HOW TO MAKE MEALTIME WORK:

HOST A POTLUCK. You can get the benefits of eating together in deceptively simple ways. Gather a few friends or families once a week (start with once a month, then increase frequency). Keep it fresh by creating fun but accessible food themes and encouraging friends to bring one new guest each time. Rotate who hosts so you don't always get stuck with the dishes.

MAKE A COMMITMENT to a group or family meal several nights a week. Treat it like anything else that is an established part of your life and you will soon create a habit. Your friends and family will, too.

TRADE PERFECTIONISM FOR CONNECTION. Don't worry about hitting some gourmet benchmark. Instead, focus on fresh, nourishing ingredients prepared simply. Go for one-pan or -pot meals (like roasting meats and veggies on a cookie sheet, using a slow cooker for soups and stews, placing ingredients on cutting boards with dipping sauces) and give your attention to the people, not the kitchen.

SHARE THE RESPONSIBILITY. Eating together takes some preparation and cleanup time. Be sure to share the duties so they don't all fall on one person. Tasty, healthy meals take some planning, so delegate tasks to all involved. Even very young kids can pitch in by setting the table. View the entire meal, from shopping to cleanup, as a shared experience. Encourage everyone to participate, and make a commitment to set down all devices throughout the process.

TAKE IT OUTSIDE. Eating in nature just feels so right. Whether it's on your city fire escape or in your local park or own backyard, enlist your crew to dine al fresco.

You can light up the BBQ or pull together a simple and delicious picnic.

MAKE IT FAMILY STYLE. Get everyone involved by serving big platters of food that must be passed around the table. Or add a DIY element to dinner with interactive, build-your-own dishes like healthy pizza or burritos with a variety of add-on toppings. Kids of all ages will run to the table!

SEEK OUT SUPPER CLUBS. If you live alone, you can still dine with others! There are many exciting pop-ups happening around the country, where aspiring and established chefs cook for mixed groups of food lovers outside of restaurant confines, including right on the farm, if you're in a rural area. (Check out outstandinginthefield. com for a gourmet farm treat.) Adventurous eaters can also gather through meet-ups to explore local dining scenes or a specific cuisine, and restaurants with communal tables can also bring individuals together. Cooking classes are another place where strangers gather around the cutting board to learn and eat together. Some quick internet research should give you some promising leads for these dining options.

Starting to bring awareness not only to what you eat, but how (and with whom) you eat, is an essential aspect of a well-rounded and happy life.

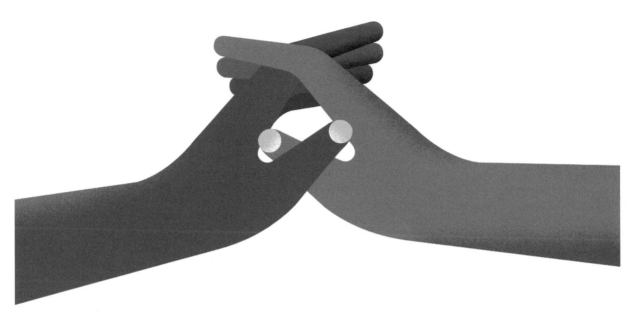

TOUCH AND BE TOUCHED

HAVE YOU BEEN TOUCHED ENOUGH TODAY? LIKELY YOU HAVE NOT; WE LIVE IN A TOUCH-DEFICIENT SOCIETY. GESTURES OF GREETING BETWEEN FRIENDS AND ACQUAINTANCES HAVE BECOME INCREASINGLY LESS PHYSICAL. FAMILY MEMBERS SPEND GREATER AMOUNTS OF TIME "TOGETHER BUT ALONE," ABSORBED IN SCREEN TIME OR

WORK. SOMETIMES, IT'S JUST NOT CLEAR *HOW* TO show care or concern with touch—what's the proper protocol? But we shouldn't let these obstacles stall us, because we suffer from this lack of contact. It's been shown that infants who are deprived of touch are at higher risk for social, emotional, and physical problems later in life and that consistent, loving touch leads to healthy brain development and the ability to sustain a robust sense of self. This need for physical affection doesn't change much just because you grow up.

When you are touched by a reassuring hand, be it from a friend or loved one, a trusted health practitioner, or even an enthusiastic dance partner, it tells your body and brain that there is social support around you. Tension can release, stress levels drop, and the immune system gets a boost to protect you from everyday viruses like colds. A firm and meaningful hug is even more effective, first because it creates a feeling of trust and safety and allows for open and honest interaction, supporting healthy relationships. Second, a good hug stimulates pressure receptors under your skin, which leads to a chain of events including increased activity of the vagus nerve, a key component of the parasympathetic nervous system, which relaxes you. It also triggers the brain to release oxytocin, and this mood-enhancing, bond-forming chemical—the key to early mother-baby attachment—also boosts your self-esteem and reduces anxiety and feelings of aloneness. By flooding you with relaxing and uplifting chemistry, a good hug can reconnect you to your feeling self—your emotional experience—which can be hard to access otherwise.

You don't have to be in a physical relationship to get more bodily contact in your life. However, if you are in one, or have a family, notice how often you and your loved ones connect through touch. It may be less than you think.

HOW TO MAKE CONTACT MORE OFTEN

- RECEIVE BODYWORK from a trusted practitioner, or, if you prefer, energy work like acupuncture (where your body is gently cared for but not overly touched). And regularly practice self-massage (page 200).

- GET A MANICURE OR PEDICURE.

- JOIN A DANCE CLASS that involves touch, from traditional partner styles like salsa to more experimental "contact dance."

- PRACTICE THOUGHTFUL TOUCH in conversation, like a hand on the arm to show you are listening deeply or a hand on the back when someone is distressed.

- COMMIT TO FIVE MEANINGFUL HUGS A DAY with your partner or family members and see how it promotes harmony (or helps smooth over discord).

- INVITE PHYSICAL PLAY WITH YOUR KIDS: piggyback rides, acrobatics and yoga, playful roughhousing.

- IF YOU ARE A NEW PARENT, engage in baby-wearing, breastfeeding, and/or co-sleeping.

- PARTICIPATE IN A PROFESSIONALLY GUIDED CUDDLE PARTY (cuddleparty.com), a safe, social, and nonsexual workshop oriented around healthy touch and communication.

- TAKE CARE OF A PET (page 215).

- LEARN HOW TO GIVE A MASSAGE and offer it to loved ones and friends.

HUG ETIQUETTE

Respecting boundaries is essential when it comes to touch. Healthy touch that feels safe and respectful to each party involves awareness of personal space, plus giving and reading body language or verbal cues to ensure the recipient wants to receive. Make direct eye contact with your intended hug-ee, offer physical cues such as outstretched arms, and, if hugging isn't already part of your friendship repertoire, include verbal cues like "Would you like a hug?"

- TRY ACROYOGA (acroyoga.org), a liberating partner-based movement practice that connects you to others through touch and movement.

- And of course . . . INVITE MORE INTIMACY and sex into your life (page 210).

Kindness is a muscle you can start to flex and that grows the more you use it.

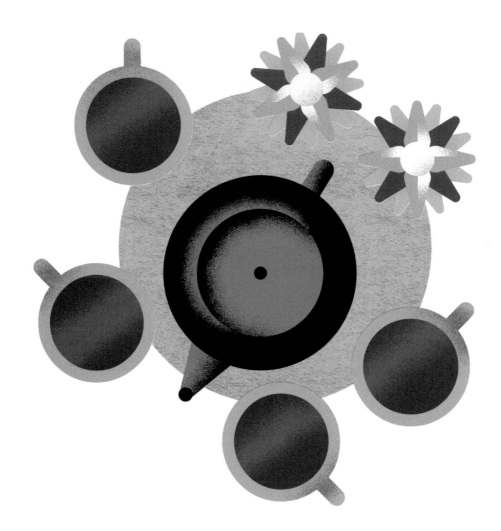

RETURN TO RITUAL

"WE HUNGER FOR BOTH COMMUNITY AND COMMUNION, THE FEELINGS FOUND IN THE CONSCIOUS PRACTICE OF RITUALS," WRITES PRACTICAL SPIRITUALITY TEACHER **BARBARA BIZIOU**, A LONGTIME FRIEND AND COL-LEAGUE, AND AUTHOR OF THE BOOK *THE JOY OF RITUAL*. BARBARA TEACHES HOW EVERYDAY OCCASIONS CAN BE

HOW TO BE WELL EXPERT

IMBUED WITH MORE MEANING TO HELP US MAKE sense of the world, expand our awareness, and connect to the great mystery of life. Humans have always woven ritual into the fabric of the everyday. Tea ceremonies were traditionally friendship rituals; a sweat lodge

was a ritual of releasing and letting go; and rites of passage, from coming of age to marriage to grieving, have long been acknowledged through rituals that connect us to the deeper story of shared human experience and make us feel comforted and held.

Small personal rituals, done on your own terms, can punctuate today's rush. They serve to slow down time, and they can tether you to a stratum of life that often gets lost in the mundane: the historic, ancestral, and timeless side of who you are. They can lend consistency and rhythm to a fractured-feeling week and enrich even a hectic day with quality. These personal rituals can be simple things that enhance your daily routines, like setting the dinner table with placemats and lit candles; creating a pre-bed wind down (page 110)—for yourself, not just your children!—or spending morning moments in contemplation, meditation, or reflective writing (page 228) before you give your energy to others.

Personal rituals can also be larger collective actions that celebrate milestones—the completion of a major project, the impending birth or adoption of a child, or the opening of a new business—or that support and honor you and others through life's big transitions. What makes any small or large action into a ritual is that it is an intentional act that momentarily shifts your consciousness from one state to another, helping you drop beyond the to-do lists and survival mode to touch something more substantial. Barbara teaches that the brain doesn't differentiate between real and symbolic acts: If you decide your shower is a ritual of purification after stress and anxiety, the brain reads it as so and your shower has helped you release and renew.

Integrating rituals into life does not have to involve fire, flowers, and song, unless you want it to. You can design your own small rituals by deciding on an intention and creating a set sequence of steps: a clear beginning, stepping away from other demands for a moment, bringing a touch or two that denotes a sacred space of some kind for the action, and an ending that allows for contemplation. Creating a sacred space can mean using your special teapot and cups, or spraying essential oils into the air during morning sun salutations. These simple things create a container for your experience, delineating it from ordinary, mundane life. One ritual Barbara is frequently asked to create for her students is a friendship ritual that helps friends foster deeper connections and forge more meaningful relationships. "By wrapping your friendship in the tenets of ritual, outside of ordinary time and space,

you'll be providing the focused opportunity that makes any relationship more likely to bloom and grow," she explains.

Here is a simple outline upon which you can build with other elements Barbara shares in her books and on her website, barbarabiziou.com.

A RITUAL FOR FRIENDSHIP

1. **GATHER A GROUP OF FRIENDS TOGETHER.** Sit in a circle. Place a bowl of beads in the center of the circle and give everyone a length of string.

2. **TURN TO THE PERSON ON YOUR LEFT** and share details that have meant the most to you regarding his or her friendship. A few examples: "Liz, you were there for me when my mother was rushed to the hospital." "Jordan, your support was crucial to me when I was in grad school." "Joanne, you always bring perspective into any situation." "Mark, you are always up for an adventure."

3. **WHEN YOU ARE FINISHED, PICK A BEAD FROM THE CENTER OF THE CIRCLE** and give it to the person you just shared with. Continue to go around the circle until you have shared with each person.

4. **THE NEXT PERSON REPEATS THE SAME RITUAL** of sharing and giving out beads, until everyone has had a turn.

5. **AT THE END OF THE RITUAL, EACH PERSON HAS A STRING OF BEADS TO MAKE A BRACELET OR NECKLACE.** You can also hang the strung beads on your wall or in your car as a symbol of your friends' support.

NEVER STOP LEARNING

SCHOOL MAY BE OUT (FOR DECADES), BUT THAT DOESN'T MEAN YOU SHOULD STOP LEARNING. WHETHER YOU'RE A NEW GRAD OR NEWLY RETIRED, THE HUMAN BRAIN IS DESIGNED TO TAKE ON NEW CHALLENGES AND EMBARK ON UNCHARTED TERRITORY THROUGHOUT YOUR LIFETIME. KEEPING YOUR GRAY MATTER ACTIVE HAS

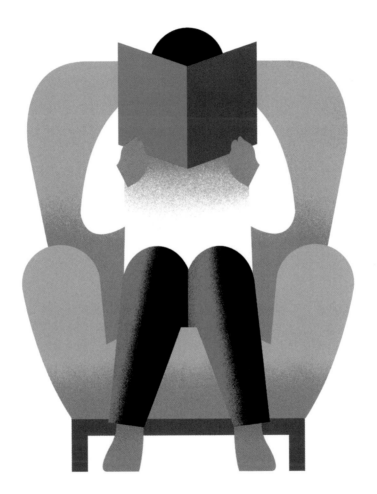

CLEAR BENEFITS. GROWING RESEARCH SHOWS THAT trying new things creates new neural pathways, which can help prevent degenerative disease like dementia while also giving your self-esteem a healthy boost. The bottom line? It feels good to grasp something new, and we're engineered to do so.

In fact, learning new things is a fundamental aspect of psychological well-being; we are wired to progress and evolve. Every time we take on the challenge of understanding a new concept, we push ourselves to grow and live a bigger life, and when we expand like this we feel inspired, capable, and more alive. There's even a term for this: *eudaimonia,* a Greek word that roughly translates to "living one's life to the fullest." Today there is more focus on eudaimonia than ever before. Researchers are discovering that stretching yourself to learn new things brings with it a greater sense of purpose and fulfillment, leading to greater happiness and health. Eudaimonia can lead to lower cortisol levels, improved immune function, and better sleep.

Thankfully, learning doesn't have to mean cramming with a textbook. If you're not the academic type—and some of the brightest folks aren't—you can stretch your brain in countless other ways. Attempting anything new will help to keep the brain juicy and activated. You can cook a new dish, walk along an unfamiliar route, or discuss a subject you've never explored before. You can also take a pottery class, try Zumba or yoga, or play a new board game with your kids. There are crossword puzzles and sudoku to keep you company on public transit, and language courses and TED talks to get your brain moving while driving (or stuck in traffic).

If you're intimidated to try something new, worried that you'll look silly in that hip-hop class or sound awkward in that Portuguese course, remember that learning new things requires you to be catapulted out of your comfort zone. It is in that slightly uncomfortable space that you step into more of who you are and meet new parts of yourself. This exploration can be a refreshing antidote to the repetitive grind that comprises so much of modern life. When you make the time to get to your weekly macramé (or knitting, jewelry-making, or glass-blowing) class, you are stepping outside of your everyday self, pushing past established roles and identities. When you make time to learn something new, you become so much more than your duties and responsibilities—more than parent, employee, or spouse. You become curiosity and possibility.

While it's wonderful to commit to a structured class that meets in person (there's nothing wrong with online courses, but you can't beat the collective energy created from a roomful of people all learning something together), learning doesn't have to have a syllabus. Following the Buddhist concept of *beginner's mind,* every moment is an opportunity to learn and grow; some spiritual traditions even believe we are reborn in every minute. For example, you can decide to see the people in your everyday life with fresh eyes: Instead of expecting friends, colleagues, or family members to act a certain way, allow them to surprise you by refusing to put them in a box. You can view everything in your life with an untainted beginner's mind. Try and see what happens.

COMMIT TO LEARNING SOMETHING NEW EACH WEEK:

IF YOU COMMUTE TO WORK, TAKE A NEW ROUTE or a new form of transportation

SIGN UP FOR AN ART OR CRAFTING CLASS in an area you have never explored before (drawing, painting, sculpture, graphic design, knitting, etc.)

JOIN (OR START!) A BOOK CLUB

START A COOKING CLUB (make one new recipe every other week or once a month)

STUDY A NEW LANGUAGE; look for classes at a local college or university

TAKE A WALK OR A HIKE in an unfamiliar neighborhood or on a trail that is brand-new to you

TEACH YOURSELF DIY HOME IMPROVEMENTS (YouTube can be a great ally here)

EXPERIMENT WITH GARDENING

TAKE A WRITING OR PUBLIC SPEAKING CLASS

ASK YOUR CHILD TO TEACH YOU SOMETHING NEW (a joke, a dance, a complicated handshake)

WRITE YOUR WAY BACK TO YOURSELF

WRITING IS ONE OF THE MOST EFFECTIVE, AND AFFORDABLE, METHODS OF MENTAL AND EMOTIONAL SELF-
CARE. THE SIMPLE ACT OF PLACING YOUR THOUGHTS ON THE PAGE HELPS IMMENSELY WITH PROCESSING CHALLENGING EMOTIONS, WORKING OUT COMPLEX PROBLEMS, SPARKING CREATIVITY, AND BRINGING IDEAS

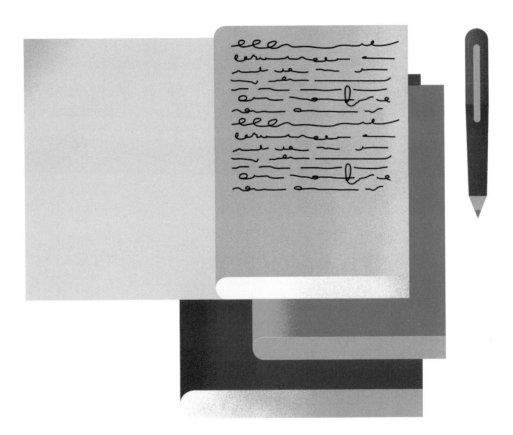

TO LIFE. YOU CAN CALL IT JOURNALING, FREE WRITING, or expository writing—the name is not important, and the method isn't, either. This kind of writing is completely yours, a personal, private, and intimate process that is between just you and the page. You don't have to be an English major or a connoisseur of fine literature to write your way back to yourself. All you need is a pen, a blank piece of paper, and the desire to learn more about yourself or to find some relief from heavy feelings.

The aim here is not to write a perfectly honed essay. In this case, even grammar takes a backseat as you use the process of putting pen to paper to unearth subconscious emotions, get a new perspective on a relationship or situation, or create some real estate in a mind, and heart, that may be swirling with thoughts, questions, or ideas. Writing freely, with no editing, sculpting, or judging, can lead you to some genuine epiphanies and help you release pent-up emotions. If left unaddressed these emotions can lodge inside us, taking up space, sapping us of energy, or even making us sick. Many people find that they sleep better after journaling, as the pestering thoughts live on the page instead of jostling around in their heads all night. Writing freely and honestly may take some practice at first, but when you get the hang of it, you may be surprised at what truths spill onto the page.

Your writing is yours alone, but you don't have to do it alone. There are excellent tools available to help you get started or to lean on. A classic and timeless free-writing device is author Julia Cameron's "Morning Pages" from her book *The Artist's Way*. You can also receive daily writing prompts in your inbox from figment.com or use an online journaling tool like 750words.com. Write in the way that feels best to you, but note that there's something special about writing with a pen. According to Julia Cameron, it's because it connects you to yourself in a deeper way as your brain slows down to match the speed of your hand.

Free writing, whether by keyboard or hand, also triggers the unconscious mind, where all the good stuff (or real stuff) is stored. Writing in this way, with no set goal or editing, is a therapeutic process that can be deeply cathartic and enlightening.

HOW TO DO IT:

Any amount of free writing will be beneficial, but you'll get the most out of it if you come up with a realistic writing commitment. This can look like five to ten minutes each morning before getting out of bed, or twenty minutes before going to sleep at night. Whatever time you choose, commit to it.

To begin, start writing whatever is crossing your consciousness in that moment: a feeling, a gripe, a dream, an anxiety. Ritual expert and Be Well pro Barbara Biziou suggests using three key phrases and writing to each: "I feel . . ." "I need . . ." "I want . . ."

Once you start, keep writing for all the time allotted, even if you are bored or antsy (write about being bored and antsy!). Just keep your hand moving—it allows your unconscious mind to loosen up and reveal what it's holding. Don't correct spelling, don't edit, don't worry about punctuation.

When time is up, put your pen down. Biziou suggests ending with the question "What do I need to know right now?" in order to connect with your inner knowing, and you'll soon find that you won't need to ask yourself. What you "need to know" might very well come spilling out onto the page and surprise you with its insight.

You don't have to be an English major or a connoisseur of fine literature to write.

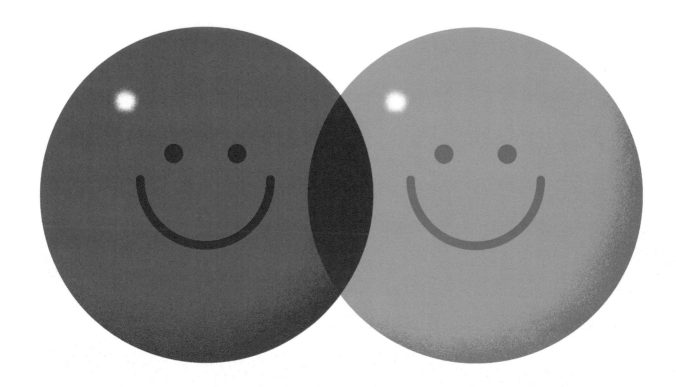

INVEST IN **FRIENDSHIP**

AS A CHILD AND YOUNG ADULT, FRIENDSHIPS WERE AN EXPECTED PART OF YOUR LIFE. BUOYED BY THE SHARED EXPERIENCE OF SCHOOL AND NOT YET BURDENED BY THE PRESSURES OF ADULT LIFE (CARING FOR A FAMILY, PAYING BILLS, BUILDING A CAREER), YOU WERE FREE TO NURTURE DEEP AND MEANINGFUL CONNECTIONS

WITH OTHERS. AS YOU AGE, YOUR PRIORITIES OFTEN shift, yet your need for gratifying friendship doesn't fade away. About 20 percent of people struggle with too much alone time, and a third of Americans aged over forty-five say they are lonely.

It makes sense that we long for companionship. Genuine and lasting friendships are a key part of a fulfilling life, shown to improve health and increase longevity by boosting optimism and connection. Trusting that someone has your back in good times and bad actually helps you live longer. But real friendship isn't a given as a busy, responsibility-laden adult, when it can be challenging to find friends who really understand you or to make the time to grow an acquaintance into a true friend. Hectic schedules, frequent moves, and major life changes can push friendships to the wayside. The upside? It's never too late to make new friends.

HERE'S HOW TO MAKE NEW FRIENDS:

1 Start with a clear intention. It won't happen unless you really want it to.

2 Take a friendship-making step each week. This may include going to an event, striking up a conversation with someone intriguing, or following up with a friendship that has faded. You can also venture into the new realm of online "friend dating" through dating apps like Bumble, which lets you connect with potential platonic pals through its BFF feature.

3 Be proactive. If you feel a connection with someone, take it to the next level. Invite him or her to have coffee, over for dinner, or to take a hike.

4 Follow up. If you meet someone you like, go with the momentum. Follow up quickly with an invitation or start another conversation. Yes, it's kind of like dating.

5 Say yes. If someone invites you out, say yes! Friendships don't happen while you're snuggled in bed watching Netflix.

6 Avoid small talk. To spark meaningful conversation (the heart of every real friendship), trade "What do you do?" for "What do you care about?"

7 Become a stellar listener. Trust and intimacy are grown from feeling heard. When a new friend speaks, really listen.

8 Go on adventures together. Shared experiences are deeply bonding, especially when they involve challenges.

9 Find a shared interest and community. Many friendships are born from yoga studios and gym classes. The website atletosports.com connects you to other athletes looking to play a sport or do an activity. Show up regularly enough to a studio, match, or trail, and you're bound to connect with others.

10 Get creative. Maybe your pet can make the intros for you! Meet My Dog helps you and your dog socialize together—ball chasing for the pets, a chat and exercise for the owners—so both of you can boost your social lives and make new friends.

11 Don't take things personally. Rejection is part of the process. If a potential new friend declines an invitation, it doesn't mean you're not a good person. It may simply mean that he or she does not have the space for developing a new relationship right now.

>>

Genuine and lasting friendships are a key part of a fulfilling life.

<<

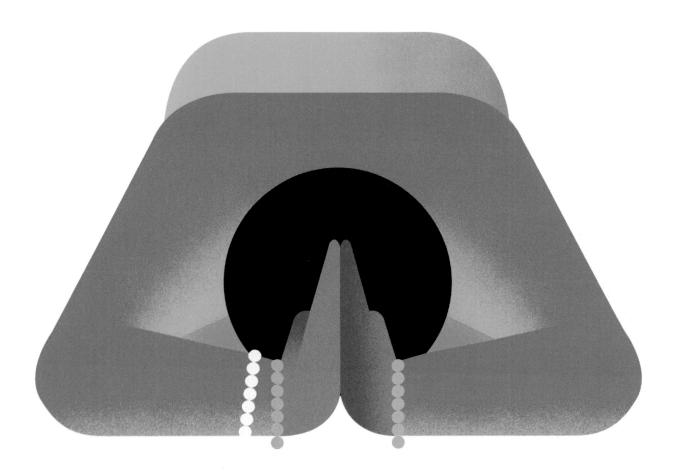

COUNT YOUR **BLESSINGS**

THIS IS GRATITUDE'S MOMENT—NEVER BEFORE HAS THE TERM RECEIVED SUCH AIRPLAY. IT'S SPLASHED ACROSS THE COVERS OF SELF-HELP BOOKS, EMBLAZONED ON WRITING JOURNALS, AND HASHTAGGED ON SOCIAL MEDIA POSTS. AND NEVER BEFORE HAVE WE NEEDED IT SO BADLY. WE LIVE IN A TIME OF POLITICAL

UPHEAVAL, CHRONIC DEPRESSION AND ANXIETY, AND incessant striving for more. Peace, contentment, and happiness can seem unrealistic or simply unattainable. Gratitude is a way out.

Gratitude is the practice of turning your attention to the goodness that is already in your life. This isn't a complex philosophy reserved for the spiritual elite; it's a simple but powerful way to reframe your perspective on life. When you view your world through a thankful lens, more good things start to happen. Researchers have found that gratitude contributes to more positive emotions, a deeper enjoyment of good experiences, increased ability to navigate difficult circumstances, better health, and stronger relationships. As a clinician, I have been struck many times by the way that patients who are grateful for something in their lives tend to handle health problems more smoothly and rebound from illness more easily.

Appreciating good things sounds easy enough, but gratitude is a practice because it takes practice. Without awareness, our worldview shifts easily to the negative. We take inventory of our lives and what's missing or imperfect seems to stand out in shining neon colors, while the good stuff fades to the background. When you practice gratitude, you make a conscious decision to feel satisfied with what you have instead of longing for what you don't. Like any new practice, you strengthen your gratitude muscles by using them, directing them to a new way of working until it becomes habitual.

The foundation of the gratitude philosophy is that each moment of each day presents you with an opportunity to be appreciative for something. That said, seeing the positive doesn't mean that you pretend that something is good when it's actually hurtful or challenging. The goal is not to forcefully transform yourself into a Pollyanna. Instead you are training yourself to see the good that actually exists around or alongside the challenge, and to notice the ripple effect of this positive perspective: One positive thought very often triggers another.

Practicing gratitude will positively influence your life only if you integrate it into your daily life.

HERE'S HOW TO DO IT:

MAKE A COMMITMENT TO PRACTICE GRATITUDE. You will be on the gratitude train, and then you'll inevitably fall off. You'll find yourself complaining or comparing yourself to others, and then you'll stop and return to thankfulness. This will happen over and over. Your commitment to practicing gratitude will bring you back each time.

KEEP A GRATITUDE JOURNAL. This can be as simple as a quick list dashed off before sleep each night or it can be a lengthier recounting of the positive things, feelings, and experiences that crossed your path during the day. Nothing is too big or too small. You may have passed a beautiful flower on the way to work or indulged in a delicious bit of dark chocolate after lunch. You may have nailed the presentation or shared a sweet moment with your child at bedtime. There is always a moment of goodness. You just have to look for it.

RECITE GRATITUDE PRAYERS. Many spiritual traditions include prayers of gratitude. You can make up your own and recite it upon waking and before sleeping. Simply express your gratitude for the gifts that are in your life, such as your health, loved ones, home, financial security, creative expression, and career opportunities. You can express gratitude for anything and everything that is positive, and you can even be grateful for the gifts that are yet to come with this simple affirmation: "I am grateful for unknown blessings already on their way."

In times of turmoil, gratitude is a way out.

FIND YOUR TRIBE

THE CALL TO GATHER IS GETTING LOUDER. IT'S HEARD IN THE RISE OF MUSIC, YOGA, AND ARTS FESTIVALS WHERE PARTICIPANTS CAMP OUT *EN FAMILLE* FOR SEVERAL DAYS, AND WORKSHOPS WHERE PEOPLE TRADE SKILLS AND TEACH CLASSES. ON ONE END OF THE SPECTRUM, IT'S SEEN IN THE INCREASE OF CIRCLES FOR THE

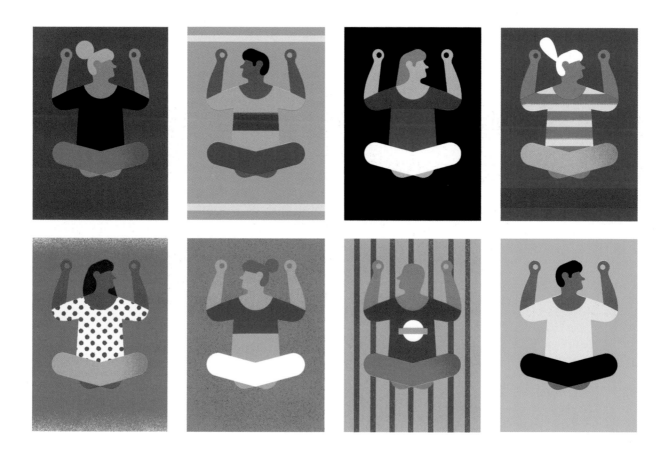

FULL MOON OR SOLSTICE, AND ON THE OTHER END, team obstacle racing over rigorous terrain; both are examples of individuals gathering for authentic experiences as a clan. This gathering spirit is evident in a more mainstream way in the growth of meet-ups, where once-strangers come together around shared interests like healthy cooking or hiking, not to mention the boom in activism and marching for a cause. It's even seen in the return of home-sharing after decades of solitary and nuclear-family living.

I think this collective urge to find a tribe is a growing backlash against the isolating effects of our hyper-technological existence. We want real community, the kind where others share your dreams, help bear some of your pains, and will pick you up at 2:00 a.m. when your car breaks down. For some people, that comes automatically from extended family, but for many it does not.

Finding a tribe is not quite the same thing as going on group vacations or nights out with your friends. It involves coming together for shared experiences that require effort and commitment, often oriented around a shared goal or mission. It involves a level of *interdependence,* in which individuals rely on each other to meet basic needs, and consistency, going beyond flash-in-the-pan experiences and engaging with the same folks numerous times. And a tribe typically involves a level of challenge because the glue that creates real bonds requires vulnerability and some discomfort, and genuine need for giving and receiving. The best kind of tribe includes intergenerational bonding, in which children and elders are part of the blend, for out of this comes connections that can last over time.

How can you find or make a tribe? It starts by shaking up your habits. Make the effort to step beyond your ordinary stomping grounds and go to where tribes are forming. Commit to driving to that festival or fair even though it's far and you're not sure about those porta-potties; join a group at a wellness or educational retreat or an herbal conference where you learn about healing plants; get a group together for wilderness trips or join outdoors groups (page 216)—or circle up with other parents coming together to collectively meet childcare needs (which can be equally wild). Try out different local interest groups through meetup.com; find a movement practice that moves you (page 119); or get more involved with a meditation group, a church, temple, or mosque, or another spiritual group that appeals. Volunteer on community projects that involve commitment and creating something together. And then when you're tired of committing to your fledgling tribe, take a rest, but don't quit. Come back and do it all again.

**PICK YOUR STYLE:
A SMORGASBORD OF TRIBAL
INSPIRATION**

What kind of tribe floats your boat? Let this eclectic mix deliver a little inspiration.

WANDERLUST.COM/FESTIVALS

FAMILYFORESTFEST.COM

OUTWARDBOUND.ORG

TOUGHMUDDER.COM

REDTENTTEMPLEMOVEMENT.COM

WOMENSHERBALCONFERENCE.COM

IC.ORG (FELLOWSHIP FOR INTENTIONAL COMMUNITY)

DAYBREAKER.COM

The best kind of tribe includes intergenerational bonding.

BE OF SERVICE

IN MY NATIVE SOUTH AFRICA, THE PHILOSOPHY OF UBUNTU IS A FOUNDATIONAL PILLAR OF LIFE. *UBUNTU* MEANS "WHAT MAKES US HUMAN IS THE HUMANITY WE SHOW EACH OTHER." IN THE U.S., WE DON'T HAVE A SINGLE PHRASE THAT CAPTURES THE SAME THING, BUT THE WORD *SEVA*, WHICH COMES FROM YOGIC

PHILOSOPHY AND MEANS "SELFLESS SERVICE FOR the good of the collective," alludes to the same thing. When you give your time, energy, and effort to a cause from a place of genuine altruism—giving for the pure sake of service to another—you experience an increased sense of belonging and connection, a greater experience of "shared humanity" that, in today's polarized culture, can be hard to find. You also get a way to be part of a solution in a world that can seem filled with paralyzing problems.

On a physiological level, volunteering and helping others has been found to correlate with higher levels of health and decreased mortality in older populations; it also generates self-esteem while reducing the incidence of stress and depression. The benefits, researchers theorize, come from an enhanced purpose in life: You are giving yourself to a cause you feel strongly about. I'd conjecture it's even bigger than that. Assisting others, especially in your local community, helps you understand and empathize with the people you live with and the place where you live, so you feel more rooted. It can connect you to people you never would have met, bestowing a richer experience of daily life. And it can let you use your skills to achieve shared goals, which feeds personal satisfaction and a sense of meaning. Today, one of the main avenues for volunteering is through initiatives in the workplace, which give partic-

ipants an opportunity to bond and find greater purpose in their work. What helps volunteering become a habit is participating in actions that are effective—for example, projects that address an important but underserved need with simple and scalable solutions—and that let you see or experience the results of your efforts.

An act of seva can be small, like walking dogs at the animal shelter or humane society, delivering meals to the elderly, or helping in urban cleanups near your home, or it can be a life-changing trip to build houses or sanitation facilities much farther afield. To find the right match for your passions and skills, start by asking friends about their experiences and find out if your workplace has any volunteer initiatives you can join; yoga studios in your area might also offer service opportunities or group trips. Your local United Way office, easily found online, will be a hub for volunteer opportunities, and the websites dosomething.org and createthegood.org share ideas for actions you can take and initiatives to join, while greatnonprofits.org lets you evaluate nonprofits based in your area. Your personal form of volunteering could start with a simple act of kindness in your immediate community, like inviting anyone in need of company and a good meal to a humble, healthy supper, cooked with love.

Helping others has been found to correlate with higher levels of health.

CELEBRATE SMALL VICTORIES

AS YOU TRAVEL THE ROAD TO BETTER HEALTH, DON'T GET CAUGHT UP IN IDEALS. IT IS TEMPTING TO PURSUE "HEALTH" LIKE THE HOLY GRAIL AND BELIEVE THAT IF YOU NAIL THE PERFECT DIET, MIX OF SUPPLEMENTS, RELATIONSHIP, AND JOB, EVERYTHING IN YOUR BODY WILL FUNCTION BRILLIANTLY AT ALL TIMES AND YOU'LL

NEVER HAVE AN OFF DAY. IRONICALLY, THIS ANXIOUS pursuit of perfection can be a hindrance to getting and staying healthy because it denies the reality of nature: Health is a dynamic state, constantly changing and in flux, and it is different for each person. There is no "perfect point" of guaranteed balance, and striving for it can drive you crazy.

There is a certain letting-go required when it comes to health. Become as aware as you can, make the best choices that are within your reach, and seek genuine support, but then relax a bit and let the changes you are initiating begin to do their work of restoring balance and resilience. In other words, get out of your own way. Jumping around from one approach to the next—so popular today—can be counterproductive and only cause more confusion and stress. And release some of the extremely high standards you might have, because you can easily self-sabotage when the changes you want do not occur at the speed or in the sequence you anticipate, or look exactly as you intended.

So, be sure to acknowledge the small successes you experience as you make shifts to better health. Make a note of what *is* working, and of what *is* changing in your experience, even if those things are very small, such as enjoying the feeling of being up early, discovering a love for freshly made green soup, or finding ten minutes of movement easier today than yesterday. Celebrate the incremental changes daily, because incremental changes add up to progress.

And if you are starting from a place that seems overwhelmingly challenging, I invite you to look at where you are through new glasses: See illness or imbalance as a message for change, an invitation to stop doing the things that aren't working, and start on a new path and a whole new way of life. When your mind comes on board with that point of view, with an attitude of compassion for yourself, the first step of true healing can occur.

Many of my patients have told me that, in retrospect, a state of poor health turned out to be a catalyst for learning deeply about who they are, what matters to them, what gives meaning to their lives, and how they can express that fully. Holding this perspective doesn't make meeting the challenges easier, but it can, over time, help them to make more sense.

Celebrate the incremental changes daily, because incremental changes add up to progress.

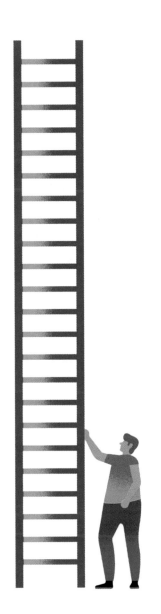

PURSUE PURPOSE, BUT DON'T CHASE BLISS

THE COMMON DENOMINATOR AMONG SOME OF THE longest-living and most vital people I have treated is that they live with purpose. They stay connected to a personal motivation that guides them as they meet the demands and challenges of life—they feel tethered to a role, an identity, or a set of activities that feel meaningful to themselves and their community—and this literally gives them something to live for.

Finding personal motivation or purpose does not happen overnight, however, and often it's neither headline-worthy nor flashy. It doesn't (usually) come from an overnight "aha!" or life-changing job; it grows over time from a commitment to a certain way of being present to life, with all its ups and downs, twists and turns. "Purpose" is a hot-button word today, when under-forties in particular are driven by a hunger for meaning in work and life, and when it can sometimes appear—at least online—as if everyone in the world has created a path ablaze with personal mission.

I asked one of my favorite—and most self-motivated—New York entrepreneurs, **Jason Wachob,** to share his thoughts on living with purpose. Jason is the founder of the wellness empire mindbodygreen.com and a definite pro when it comes to knowing how to be well.

HOW TO BE WELL EXPERT

So many people today are searching for a purposeful life and that is a really good thing! But we have become so used to having something *now* that we have gotten out of balance. We're in the age of instant gratification. If I want food I can get it in ten minutes; if I want something from Amazon, I can get it tomorrow. This leaves a lot of people hopping around in the search for meaning—jumping from one experience to the next, or from one job to the next, seeking the *"I found my purpose!"* moment, but ultimately feeling frustrated and even quite lost. Because all that moving around, and restless seeking, can be a form of busyness and distraction. It doesn't lead to depth of experience and satisfaction.

What I've discovered in my own journey, which has had numerous starts and stops and has required constant recommitment, is that purpose is not something you arrive at all of a sudden, unless you're quite lucky. For most of us, there is no crystal ball or sudden realization. The sense of purpose dawns and strengthens from the little actions you make and the choices that influence how you show up for your life each day. It's not about expecting to feel personal bliss every day or absolute fulfillment—what I call the unicorn-and-rainbows idea of purpose. It's about spending time on small things that are important to you.

The way I stay connected to purpose is to start my day with a personal practice. Right after waking, I do twenty minutes of meditation—it's nonnegotiable for me. Then I take a few moments for gratitude, whether it's for my health, wife, daughter, mother, colleagues. This sets me up for what comes. It adds a sense of purpose to why I'm here and what I'm doing, no matter where the day takes me and whether it is a good day or a tough one.

A PRACTICE OF PURPOSE

Cultivating personal purpose begins by asking yourself, "What lights me up?" First thing in the morning, take a moment to scan the day that is about to come. What small moment offers an experience of contentment today? It might be the most trivial thing, like dropping your child off at school, taking a walk with a coworker, or picking out greens at the market. Then, when these moments happen, acknowledge how these actions make you *feel* in body and mind—grounded, capable, connected to others, appreciated, loving, or beloved—these are all facets of meaning and purpose! This small mindfulness practice will nurse seeds of meaning that grow and deepen over time. They foster that "lit-up" state of vitality that purposeful people radiate—a cornerstone of longevity and health.

Purpose is not discovered. Instead, it comes from following your passions and interests, and spending time on the small things that are important to you.

MORE EXPERIENCES, FEWER THINGS

WHEN IT COMES TO THE PURSUIT OF HAPPINESS, PSYCHOLOGY RESEARCH SAYS THAT REAL-LIFE EXPERIENCES DELIVER LONGER-LASTING SATISFACTION THAN MATERIAL GOODS. WHEN PEOPLE MAKE MAJOR PURCHASES, STUDIES SHOW THEY INITIALLY REPORT HAPPINESS AKIN TO SOME OF THEIR BEST IN-PERSON EXPERIENCES LIKE

TRAVEL, CONCERTS, AND GET-TOGETHERS WITH LOVED ones. Over time, however, the satisfaction with the object fades, while happiness about experiences increases. This is because the mind "adapts" to the object and it loses its exciting veneer, and you may even start to compare the object to what other people have and find it comes up short. Conversely, the recollections of an experience, the tales you tell about it, and the relationships that grow from it become a meaningful part of the story of your life,

which delivers a deeper satisfaction; revisiting it through memory or conversation can rekindle the happy feelings.

So, spend your extra cash on doing and being, and put a little less into having. Just remember to really be present in the experience and forget about taking selfies. You'll remember more when you're fully engaged and noticing every detail with your eyes, ears, and fine senses than if you get wrapped up trying to document everything.

Feelings of contentment are more likely to come from places and experiences, rather than from objects. So spend your extra cash on doing and being, and put a little less into having.

MAKE SPACE FOR MORE FUN

BEING AN ADULT IS SERIOUS BUSINESS, ESPECIALLY WHEN YOU ARE LIVING IN SERIOUS TIMES. HOWEVER, THAT'S ALL THE MORE REASON TO MAKE SPACE FOR CAREFREE AND UNSELFCONSCIOUS FUN. NOT ONLY DOES IT LET YOU STRETCH YOUR WINGS PHYSICALLY AND MENTALLY, HAVING FUN ENCOURAGES SURPRISE, CURIOSITY,

AND CREATIVITY TO FLOW—IT RELEASES STRESS AND triggers the release of feel-good endorphins. Fun also helps you to bond with more deeply others: Many a long-lasting friendship has been built on a foundation of silly adventures and goofing around.

Fun exists purely for its own sake and has no greater purpose than to connect you to joy. Watch animals frolic, roll in dirt, or chase each other, yapping and prancing—or for that matter, watch small children do similar. The desire to engage freely in spontaneous activities that make you feel gleeful is natural and innate. But why do we do so little of it as we age? We get caught in the belief that responsibility should trump frivolity. I recommend rethinking that and making a weekly fun date of some kind a high priority, because an hour of fun can do more for your well-being than many a well-intentioned, and furrow-browed, health intervention.

A fun date can be as simple as a living room dance party (with yourself or others); a wild game of paddle ball on the beach or horseshoes at the park; or a rambunctious game of tag at the playground with your children. It could be seeing a comedy show with friends, a night doing an unusual group activity like painting or throwing pottery, or a high-energy game night for all ages. Or it could be something totally kooky that nobody but you could dream up but that makes you shine from the inside out. Most of us know *something* that our kidlike self still registers as pure fun, if we would only let that self speak.

Ironically, unless you program it in your calendar—it's Sunday morning, time to dance!—your responsible self might conspire to make you forget the commitment and stay in "productive" mode. Overrule that urge by having one or two fun coconspirators (of any age) in your life and committing to at least one short session per week that serves absolutely no purpose but getting your fun freak on.

An hour of fun can do more for your well-being than many a well-intentioned, and furrow-browed, health intervention.

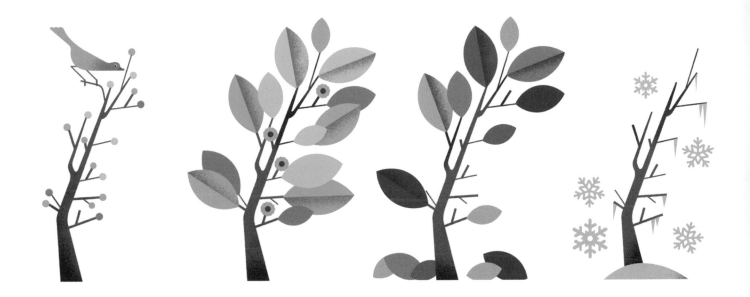

HONOR THE **SEASONS**

CHINESE MEDICINE TEACHES THAT WE ARE A MICROCOSM OF THE MACROCOSM; OUR BODIES AND OUR PSYCHES ARE INTIMATELY INFLUENCED BY THE NATURAL WORLD WE LIVE IN, ADJUSTING AND ENTRAINING TO THE RHYTHMS AND FLUCTUATIONS OF DAYTIME AND NIGHTTIME, CLIMATE, AND, OF COURSE, THE SEASONS. THESE SHIFTS

ARE SO SUBTLE THAT THEY OFTEN OCCUR BENEATH our level of awareness because we've fallen out of the custom of paying attention to them. But they occur nonetheless, and they influence how we function and feel! This is one reason that acupuncturists encourage patients to receive treatment at each change of season, to help them smoothly transition from one phase to the next. Perhaps not surprisingly, seasonal treatments aren't commonplace in the Western approach to being well.

They should be. Life today can feel strangely seasonless: Your email inbox doesn't look that different in spring versus fall; the expectations of your availability or energy levels don't change from deep winter to high summer. Within you, however, a much older and more primal clock is tracking the shifts from spring to summer and from fall to winter. When you acknowledge this innate relationship to seasons, it is like living in sync with tidal ebbs and flows: Things move more fluidly, you can anticipate times you might need extra care, and you can make sense of what you are feeling, allowing your energy, activity level, and appetite to fluctuate instead of fighting against it or insisting that you should feel the same every day of the year. Acknowledging the seasons is one very old way to know your place in the greater macrocosm that holds you—a true gift in a fragmented modern world.

One of my greatest mentors and a cherished friend and soul sister in healing is **Harriet Beinfield,** one of the foremost American educators and healers in the Chinese medical tradition, and author of *Between Heaven and Earth: A Guide to Chinese Medicine*. Here are her tips for living in line with seasonal change:

When you understand the characteristics of the seasons, you become more attuned to yourself and can harness what they offer to help you take the best care of yourself. Spring is a time of exuberant reentry after winter; you might not need as much sleep, and the world invites you to be more active outdoors—get out there, rain or shine! The renewing force of this season is strong—use it if you've been looking to make changes. You might notice a feeling of fullness, a desire to clear and reboot. Spring supports new ideas, new habits, or even a detoxifying cleanse.

Summer is a season of fun. Its longer days invite you to change up your routine and relax your schedule—look for opportunities to be unscheduled and just "be" with the birds and the bees. It's a time of pursuing frivolous delight—whenever possible, take yourself away from the to-dos. Light, fresh foods that take advantage of nature's bounty may suit you now, with a heightened ability to digest raw foods.

Fall is a time of reentry into structured rhythms, in preparation for winter. It's a time of discipline, when you want to apply your analytic skills to what's working and what's not in the ways you organize your life, and make a hierarchy of "What's most important?" to yourself, and see if you're accommodating that. In the kitchen, you may do more meal planning, stocking up of supplies, and even canning and preserving.

And as the wheel turns, and the yin season of winter calls us inward, you eat more things from under the ground, like root vegetables, and begin to make slow-cooked soups and stews and bone broths, which draw nutrition from deep within the bone. Honor the urge to slow down, be more reflective, rest, and contemplate. Practice saying no (page 197) if you want to. Winter is a time of sinking

in and of remembering that we can get off the hamster wheel of life if we choose. If new habits are harder to engrain, give yourself some space. Spring's energizing force is just around the corner.

I also suggest doing a seasonal inventory four times a year: Ask, "What was that season like for me—what am I satisfied and dissatisfied with, and what can I now reinvent? What is about to change in my environment, and how might my lifestyle shift?" Taking stock in this way, as well as honoring the seasonal shifts with solstice or equinox celebrations or just immersing yourself in nature, adds rhythm and dimension to your life. In our fast-paced world, it ensures that one season, and one year, doesn't just run on to the next.

>>

We are a microcosm of the macrocosm; our bodies and our psyches are intimately influenced by the natural world we live in.

SING!

AN AYURVEDIC HEALER ONCE TOLD ME THAT THE MOST POWERFUL TOOL FOR HEALING IS SINGING. WHEN YOU LIFT YOUR VOICE, IT RAISES YOUR SPIRITS, AND WHEN YOU FEEL TIRED, POWERLESS OR DISENFRANCHISED, THE SOUND OF YOUR OWN VOICE RINGING OUT REMINDS YOU OF YOUR AGENCY AND THE INNATE ABILITY TO

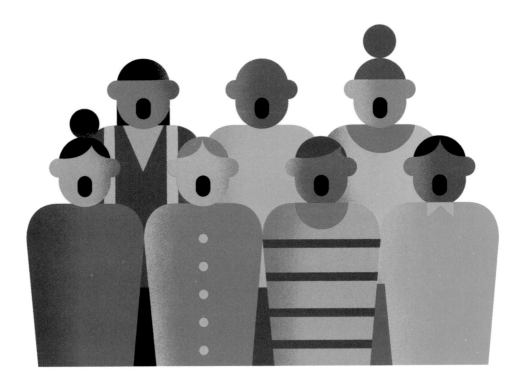

PROJECT YOURSELF INTO THE WORLD. WHEN YOU sing with others, the resonance of individual voices in harmony creates a palpable experience of wholeness, a resonance that you feel inside your body as vibrations and that transcends any belief the thinking mind may hold about being alone or inconsequential. Sing at the kitchen sink, in the car, or with the kids, or get out to karaoke. Invite friends to join for a meal with a guitar and a sing-along.

Better yet, find a group singing experience like call-and-response kirtan at a yoga studio, or a local choir or "community chorus" through meetup.com (search under "singer meetups"), and don't be shy about going alone—most people will probably be doing similar. You don't have to have a spiritual affiliation to join a choir. These days, choral groups fuse secular and sacred music, and there are even rock and pop choirs and alternative singing groups to fulfill everyone's need to sing. You can even find a cappella groups like those of Sweet Adelines International, an organization for women's barbershop singing. Give a few groups a try—if the first one isn't the right vibe, try another, until you find one where you feel in harmony. (If you'd rather play music than sing it, amateur instrumental groups exist, too.)

WHAT TO
DO WHEN . . .

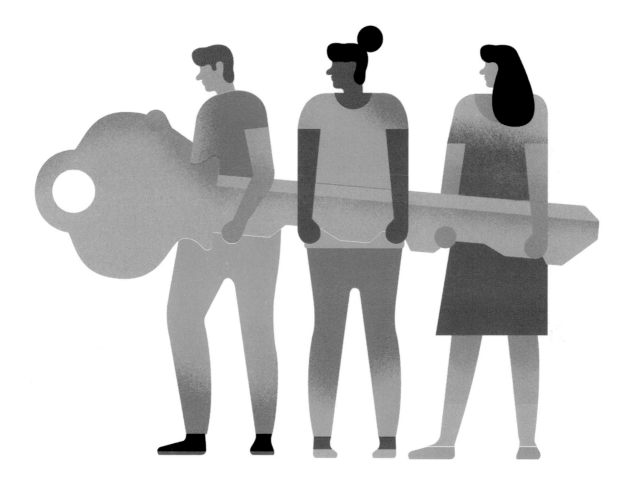

NOW THAT YOU'VE BECOME FAMILIAR WITH THE 108 how-tos that are fundamental to being well, you can start to use them in targeted ways to improve specific complaints. The following eleven strategies are my basic approaches to the most common conditions that present in my practice, and they all combine actions from the Good Medicine Mandala. For descriptions of each step, turn to the indicated pages in this book or to howtobewell.com, and use the "Boost" steps to enhance the basic steps.

While we all require individualized fine-tuning at times to completely resolve health issues, there are universal practices that I prescribe to every patient to begin repairing and resolving whatever is out of sorts. I suggest you start here, too. Consider this your troubleshooting guide of "first-line" tactics you can use to improve everyday health problems by addressing their root cause.

YOU FEEL SLUGGISH AND WANT TO REBOOT

BASIC PROTOCOL:

DO A TWO-WEEK ELIMINATION DIET to detect and remove irritating foods, page 90
EAT LOTS OF VEGETABLES, page 58
PRIORITIZE SLEEP, page 97
EXERCISE DAILY: that could mean ten-minute workouts, page 121, or a long, lazy walk, page 125
EACH DAY, PICK ONE NEW HABIT TO PRACTICE from the following:

- Spend time in nature, page 216
- Take a break from excess technology use, page 186
- Smile, Laugh, Repeat, page 205
- Sing!, page 244

BOOST:

DURING YOUR ELIMINATION DIET, ADD HERBS for addressing chronic low-grade gut infections to restore balance to the microbiome, such as berberine sulfate, black walnut hull, and grapefruit seed extract. This is what we use in the Be Well Cleanse and is described at howtobewell.com.
CLEAN OUT YOUR PANTRY of all processed foods (use Organize Your Fridge and Pantry, page 71)
PRACTICE INTERMITTENT FASTING, page 88

....

YOU WANT TO LOSE WEIGHT

BASIC PROTOCOL:

DO A TWO-WEEK ELIMINATION DIET (page 90) to detect and eliminate irritating foods, boost detoxification, and repair your gut, page 174; and see howtobewell.com for more information
QUIT SUGAR in all its forms, page 26
EAT FEWER PROCESSED FOODS, page 38
FOLLOW A LOW-CARB DIET, particularly if your blood work reveals high levels for blood sugar, HbA1c, fruc-

tosamine, and fasting insulin, page 85
PRACTICE MINDFUL EATING, page 66
EAT LOTS OF NONSTARCHY VEGETABLES, page 58
PRIORITIZE SLEEP, page 97
INCREASE STRENGTH TRAINING, page 122
PICK ONE OR TWO WAYS TO UNWIND, page 181

BOOST:

PRACTICE INTERMITTENT FASTING two or three days per week, page 88
CONSIDER A KETOGENIC PROTOCOL, page 84
WORK WITH A KNOWLEDGEABLE HEALTH PRACTITIONER (ideally one trained in functional medicine) to test the following blood markers:

- Complete metabolic panel (CMP) with lipids
- Complete blood count (CBC)
- DHEA-S
- High-sensitivity C-reactive protein (hs-CRP)
- Free testosterone
- Total testosterone
- Progesterone (for women)
- Estradiol (for women)
- Hemoglobin A1c
- Fasting insulin
- Fructosamine
- Thyroid panel (includes TSH, free T4, free T3, reverse T3, and thyroid antibodies)
- 25-hydroxy vitamin D

....

YOU ARE FREQUENTLY OVERWHELMED AND ANXIOUS

BASIC PROTOCOL:

MEDITATE DAILY (you can start with five minutes each morning), page 194
PRACTICE BREATHING EXERCISES during the day, page 184, and/or practice restorative yoga, page 206
TAKE A BREAK FROM EXCESS TECHNOLOGY (reduce social media use), page 186

SUPPLEMENT WITH ADAPTOGENS, page 67, and L-theanine, page 112
QUIT SUGAR, page 26
PRACTICE GRATITUDE, page 232
SPEND TIME IN NATURE, page 216, and practice earthing to calm the nervous system, page 161

BOOST:

REPAIR YOUR GUT—anxiety is often related to an imbalance in the gut microbiome, page 174; go to howtobewell.com for additional information
PICK ONE OR TWO WAYS TO CONNECT and do them weekly, page 213
PRACTICE SAYING NO TO OBLIGATIONS, page 197, and make time for downtime, page 198
WORK WITH A KNOWLEDGEABLE PRACTITIONER to get the following blood markers checked:

- Red blood cell magnesium
- 25-hydroxy vitamin D
- Homocysteine
- MTHFR gene mutation
- Progesterone (for women)

YOU FEEL BLOATED AND GASSY

BASIC PROTOCOL:

EAT MINDFULLY and chew well, page 66
DO A TWO-WEEK ELIMINATION DIET to detect and remove irritating foods, page 90
IF YOU ARE VEGETARIAN and eat a lot of grains and legumes, be sure to soak them to reduce lectin content, page 37
REPAIR YOUR GUT, page 174; go to howtobewell.com for additional information

BOOST:

If the above do not improve the situation, more targeted detective work is required. This could include:

- RESOLVING ANY CHRONIC LOW-GRADE INFECTIONS by working with a practitioner to determine yeast overgrowth or a parasite or bacterial infection, then using antimicrobial herbs or medication to remove them. In the case of yeast overgrowth, yeasty and fermented foods and drinks should be eliminated from your diet.
- INVESTIGATING WHETHER YOU ARE SENSITIVE TO FODMAPS, a group of foods high in a certain kind of starches that cause gas, bloating, and other GI issues. For more on this rather complex subject, see howtobewell.com.

PRACTICE YOGA, page 206, and/or gentle foam rolling, page 137, targeted to the midsection to move air through the body
MEDITATE DAILY to create calm throughout the nervous system, page 194

YOU ARE ALWAYS TIRED

BASIC PROTOCOL:

GET BLOOD WORK DONE to rule out any vitamin deficiency (especially if you are vegetarian); work with a knowledgeable practitioner to test for the following:

- Complete metabolic panel (CMP) with lipids
- Complete blood count (CBC)
- Erythrocyte sedimentation rate (ESR)
- High-sensitivity C-reactive protein (hs-CRP)
- DHEA-S
- Cortisol
- Thyroid panel (includes TSH, free T4, free T3, reverse T3, and thyroid antibodies)
- Free testosterone
- Total testosterone
- Antinuclear antibody (ANA)
- Rheumatoid factor
- Lyme disease with co-infections panel
- Epstein-Barr virus antibodies (IgG and IgM)
- MTHFR gene mutation

- Homocysteine
- Vitamins B$_{12}$, folate, and 25-hydroxy vitamin D
- Iron
- TIBC (how much iron is being utilized)
- Ferritin
- Iodine
- Red blood cell magnesium
- Selenium
- Zinc

DO A TWO-WEEK ELIMINATION DIET to detect and remove irritating foods, page 90

RESET YOUR BODY CLOCK and practice the sleep rhythm and sleep hygiene habits throughout Ring 3, page 98

EXERCISE DAILY (strength training, page 122, has been shown to be the most effective exercise for fighting chronic fatigue)

USE ADAPTOGENS to support your body during times of stress, page 67, and reduce your caffeine intake

CREATE A SMART SUPPLEMENT STRATEGY (be sure to include a multivitamin and CoQ10 for mitochondrial support), page 172

BOOST:

SPEND TIME IN NATURE, page 216, and take your shoes off, page 161

MEDITATE DAILY, page 194

PRACTICE RESTORATIVE YOGA (especially in the evening), page 206

YOU ARE CONSTIPATED

BASIC PROTOCOL:

DO A TWO-WEEK ELIMINATION DIET to detect and remove constipating foods, page 90

ADD FERMENTED FOODS AND/OR PROBIOTICS to your diet, page 54

DRINK PLENTY OF FILTERED WATER, page 154

HAVE A LIGHT OR LIQUID DINNER (such as blended soups) and finish it three hours before bedtime to rest your digestion

TAKE MAGNESIUM CITRATE or magnesium oxide nightly, page 112

IMPROVE DIGESTION by drinking 1 tablespoon apple cider vinegar mixed in water and/or bitters, page 176, before meals, and after meals, chew fennel seeds or infuse them into a tea for sipping.

EXERCISE DAILY and incorporate yoga twists and/or gentle abdominal massage (use clockwise strokes while lying down)

GET INTO A RHYTHM of moving your bowels at the same time each day; consider using a Squatty Potty for optimal ergonomics

BOOST:

IF MAGNESIUM IS NOT WORKING SUFFICIENTLY, try triphala (an Ayurvedic remedy). For acute cases, try Swiss Kriss (a senna-based herbal laxative) temporarily, but do not become dependent on it.

MEDITATE DAILY and incorporate several other Unwind actions to improve stress, page 194

>> **A physical symptom is a pointer to something in the body system that is out of balance, not an annoying disruption that must be extinguished at all costs.** <<

ADD FLAXSEEDS (and chia seeds if you tolerate them) to smoothies before blending, page 67

INCREASE THE AMOUNT OF HEALTHY FATS in your diet, page 30

TRY COLONIC HYDROTHERAPY with a trusted practitioner

INCORPORATE ANTIMICROBIAL HERBS as part of a deeper process to rebalance the gut microbiome, page 176

RULE OUT LOW THYROID FUNCTION

....

YOU HAVE HEARTBURN OR ACID REFLUX

BASIC PROTOCOL:

DO A TWO-WEEK ELIMINATION DIET to detect and remove irritating foods, page 90

FOLLOW A LOW-CARB DIET, page 85 (it improves these conditions in many cases)

ADD FERMENTED FOODS AND/OR PROBIOTICS to your diet, page 54

IMPROVE DIGESTION by drinking 1 tablespoon apple cider vinegar mixed in water and/or bitters, page 176, before meals

IF YOU ARE ON PPIs (proton pump inhibitors) for acid reflux, slowly taper off them under a doctor's supervision; do not stop cold turkey because you will get a rebound effect

LOOK FOR HEARTBURN OR GI-SUPPORTING SUPPLEMENTS containing one or all of the following nutrients, or take them individually:

- DGL (deglycyrrhizinated licorice): 400 to 800 mg 30 minutes before each meal
- Mastic gum: 250 to 500 mg 30 minutes before each meal or 1,000 mg before bed at night
- Zinc carnosine: about 75 mg per day
- Aloe vera: about 2 tablespoons per day
- Probiotic: 30–100 billlion

....

YOU KEEP GETTING SICK

BASIC PROTOCOL:

GET BLOOD WORK DONE to rule out any vitamin deficiency (especially if you are vegetarian), working with a knowledgeable practitioner to test for the following:

- Complete metabolic panel (CMP) with lipids
- Complete blood count (CBC)
- Erythrocyte sedimentation rate (ESR)
- High-sensitivity C-reactive protein (hs-CRP)
- Thyroid panel (includes TSH, free T4, free T3, reverse T3, and thyroid antibodies)
- Antinuclear antibody (ANA)
- Lyme disease with co-infections panel
- Epstein-Barr virus antibodies (IgG and IgM)
- MTHFR gene mutation
- Homocysteine
- Vitamin B_{12}
- Vitamin A
- 25-hydroxy vitamin D
- Folate
- Iron
- TIBC (how much iron is being utilized)
- Ferritin
- Selenium
- Zinc

DO A TWO-WEEK ELIMINATION DIET to detect and then remove irritating foods, page 90

ADD FERMENTED FOODS AND/OR PROBIOTICS to your diet, page 54

PRIORITIZE SLEEP, page 97, and make time for downtime during your day, page 198

ENSURE ADEQUATE VITAMIN D through sun or supplementation, page 156

DO NOT TAKE ANTIBIOTICS INDISCRIMINATELY, page 143

USE ADAPTOGENS when you're feeling stressed, page 67

USE COCONUT OIL (a natural antimicrobial) in your diet, and drink bone broth frequently (for heightened immunity), page 43

ENJOY TEAS OR TONICS made from immune-boost-

ing herbs like Andrographis, echinacea, elderberry, and astragalus
WHEN COOKING, BE LIBERAL WITH SPICES like garlic, ginger, and turmeric, page 82
CONSIDER USING EITHER YIN QIAO OR GAN MAO LING, which are classic Chinese immunity-boosting formulas (use only one, not both)

BOOST:

EXERCISE DAILY
PICK TWO OR THREE TIPS FROM UNWIND, page 181, and practice daily to reduce stress
CREATE A SMART, TARGETED SUPPLEMENT STRATEGY according to your blood test results, which includes a good multivitamin, page 172
CONSIDER DOING A FULL DETOXIFICATION CLEANSE WITH ANTIMICROBIAL HERBS to improve the condition of your gut microbiome (go to howtobewell.com)
VISIT AN INFRARED SAUNA REGULARLY, page 178

....

YOU HAVE BRAIN FOG AND CAN'T THINK AS CLEARLY AS YOU'D LIKE

BASIC PROTOCOL:

DO A TWO-WEEK ELIMINATION DIET to detect and remove irritating foods, page 90
REPAIR THE GUT, page 174; go to howtobewell.com for additional information
AUDIT YOUR MEDS, page 143; are statin drugs or other prescription drugs making you foggy?
PRIORITIZE SLEEP and reset your clock, page 97
EXERCISE DAILY, page 120
MEDITATE DAILY, page 194
TAKE TARGETED SUPPLEMENTS: In addition to vitamin D and fish oils (preferably krill oil; look for an oil that delivers about 1,000 mg of DHA), try adding a daily dose of anti-inflammatory curcumin (follow the directions on the bottle), an adaptogen like rhodiola, and alpha-lipoic acid (a powerful antioxidant that improves mitochondrial

function and frequently improves brain fog; start with 300 mg per day)

BOOST:

GET STRONG! Strength training using resistance (weights) has been shown to be more effective for mental performance than toning-type workouts, page 122
DRINK BONE BROTH frequently, page 43

....

YOU HAVE ACNE OR OTHER SKIN ISSUES

BASIC PROTOCOL:

DO A TWO-WEEK ELIMINATION DIET to detect and remove irritating foods (dairy, sugar, and processed foods are the prime offenders here), page 90; it usually takes more than two weeks to clear up poor skin, so to start seeing results, stick to the elimination diet for as long as you can
REPAIR THE GUT, page 174; go to howtobewell.com for additional information
DRINK BONE BROTH frequently, page 43
DON'T TAKE ANTIBIOTICS INDISCRIMINATELY, page 143
PROTECT YOUR SKIN ECOLOGY (and allow the skin microbiome to balance itself), page 155; this includes doing a "clean break" with your current skincare products

BOOST:

DRINK 1 TABLESPOON OF APPLE CIDER VINEGAR diluted in water before meals, and apply the same mixture to the skin topically to support skin microbiome
TAKE PROBIOTICS, page 176
PICK TWO OR THREE TIPS FROM UNWIND, page 181, for support against stress
VISIT AN INFRARED SAUNA REGULARLY to sweat out toxins and clean pores, page 178
ADD SKIN-BOOSTING COLLAGEN POWDER to smoothies, soups, and stews, page 67

....

YOUR DOCTOR SAYS YOU HAVE HIGH CHOLESTEROL

BASIC PROTOCOL:

LEARN THE BIG PICTURE OF CHOLESTEROL—why it is essential for living, why it is actually a poor marker for health and certainly not the "be-all and end-all" of your test results, and why lowering it may not always be a good thing—at howtobewell.com.

ASK YOUR DOCTOR TO DIG DEEPER, especially if you have a family history of heart disease or other risk factors. Ask her or him to look at inflammation biomarkers, including high-sensitivity C-reactive protein (hs-CRP), fibrinogen and Lp-PLA2, Lipid Subfractionation (measures particle sizes of the LDL cholesterol), apolipoprotein B and lipoprotein(a), homocysteine level, an omega profile, red blood cell magnesium level, and genotype tests (which help determine hereditary risk). These measurable physical clues will help fill in a few more pieces of the puzzle and enable you and your doctor to develop a more customized program to help manage your risk, with or without cholesterol drugs. If your doc's not interested in looking under the medical hood, then it may be time to switch to a new mechanic.

COMMIT TO A LOW-CARB DIET (perhaps the most important action you can take), page 85; as you transition to this way of eating, be sure to eliminate all sugar from your diet (page 26), eat lots of leafy green and cruciferous vegetables (page 58) instead of starchy or root vegetables, eat healthy fats (page 30), avoid low-fat processed foods, practice composing the Perfect Plate (page 23) at each meal, and audit your oils (page 76)

EXERCISE DAILY, page 120
PRIORITIZE SLEEP, page 97
ADD THE FOLLOWING SUPPLEMENTS:

- Krill oil: 2 or 3 g per day
- CoQ10: 200 mg per day
- Magnesium: 300 to 500 mg per day
- Bergamot (the supplement, not the aromatic oil): 1 mg per day
- Niacin: Start at 250 mg per day and increase the dose by 250 mg every couple of weeks until you reach a max of 750 to 1,000 mg per day. Otherwise, niacin can cause unwanted flushing.

BOOST:

MEDITATE DAILY to help lower inflammation (by reducing cortisol), page 194
VISIT AN INFRARED SAUNA REGULARLY if possible, page 178

ACKNOWLEDGMENTS

CREATING THIS BOOK HAS BEEN EXHILARATING AND challenging, and the most collaborative book I've written yet. I am deeply indebted to the "village" of people who brought *How to Be Well* to life.

I could not have written this book without the remarkable and skilled Amely Greeven. She always understands, always hits the nail on the head, is brilliant with language and concepts, and made me sound way cooler than I really am. She gets it, she really gets it.

It was important to me that this book appeal across generations, and particularly to millennials. Not being a millennial myself, that meant I needed to enlist a team that could relate to our current culture. My right-hand woman and health coach at BeWell, Amanda Carney, brought life, light, and organization to *How to Be Well*. She is unflappable, always friendly, and warm-hearted, not to mention brilliant and knowledgeable. She helped build the dream team that made it all happen—starting with Panos Galanopoulos, Dave Schnapper, and the rest of the design team at PG&Co who made this book look as fantastic as it does. They found our illustrator Giacomo Bagnara and worked with him every step of the way, bringing the concepts to life through art and design. Giacomo's skilled work throughout speaks for itself—we were so fortunate to have him on the team.

My longtime book agent Stephanie Tade had a ball with this book from the very start. Her support, guidance, and friendship never waver.

Sincere thanks to Deb Brody, my brilliant editor, who stayed calm even when the waters got rough (hint: illustrated books with a lot of strongly opinionated people involved can be challenging). Deb, my gratitude for always standing up for what was best for the book and keeping your eye on the prize. Thank you.

To Heidi Krupp and staff for their enthusiasm for the messages in this book, and for helping spread those messages far and wide.

Fair to say I couldn't do any of this without my stellar and loyal staff at the Eleven Eleven Wellness Center, who run the practice like clockwork and make life so much easier for me.

To my daughter, Alison, and her husband, Zach, for keeping me real and always willing to be brutally honest with their feedback. Really!

My incredible wife, Janice, who for more than forty years has put up with me, supported me, loved me, and been my greatest ally.

And finally to my patients who constantly teach me and inspire me to find ways to make the world a happier and healthier place for all.

INDEX